Philosophy of Mental Disorder

This book offers an ability-based view of mental disorders. It develops a detailed analysis of the concept of inability that is relevant in the psychiatric and psychotherapeutic context by drawing on the most recent literature on the concepts of ability, reasons, and harm.

What is it to have a mental disorder? This book contends that an individual has a mental disorder if and only if (1) they are—in the relevant sense—unable to respond adequately to their available (apparent) reasons in their thinking, feeling, or acting, and (2) they are harmed by the condition underlying or resulting from that inability. The author calls this the "Rehability View." This view can account for what is "mental" about mental disorders: it is the rational relations among an individual's attitudes and actions that are "disordered," and the relevant norms are the norms of reasons. This view is compatible with explanations of mental disorders in terms of biological dysfunctions, without reducing the former to the latter. The aim is not to offer just another conception of mental disorder, but to develop a systematic approach that incorporates insights from the philosophy of psychiatry and adjacent philosophical disciplines.

Philosophy of Mental Disorder will be of interest to scholars and advanced students working in philosophy of psychiatry, philosophy of mind, philosophy of action, ethics, and mental health.

Sanja Dembić is a researcher at the "Human Abilities" Centre for Advanced Studies in the Humanities in Berlin. Her paper "Defining Addictive Disorder: Abilities Reconsidered" (Philosophers' Imprint 2021) won the Prize for Philosophy and Ethics in Psychiatry and Psychotherapy 2021 by the German Association for Psychiatry, Psychotherapy and Psychosomatics (DGPPN).

Routledge Studies in Contemporary Philosophy

For more information about this series, please visit: www.routledge.com/Routledge-Studies-in-Contemporary-Philosophy/book-series/SE0720

Philosophy of Mental Disorder

An Ability-Based Approach

Sanja Dembić

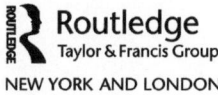
Routledge
Taylor & Francis Group

NEW YORK AND LONDON

First published 2024
by Routledge
605 Third Avenue, New York, NY 10158

and by Routledge
4 Park Square, Milton Park, Abingdon, Oxon, OX14 4RN

Routledge is an imprint of the Taylor & Francis Group, an informa business

Library of Congress Cataloging-in-Publication Data
Names: Dembić, Sanja, author.
Title: Philosophy of mental disorder : an ability-based approach / Sanja Dembić.
Description: New York, NY : Routledge, 2024. | Series: Routledge studies in contemporary philosophy | Includes bibliographical references and index.
Identifiers: LCCN 2023025445 (print) | LCCN 2023025446 (ebook) | ISBN 9781032435466 (hardback) | ISBN 9781032435473 (paperback) | ISBN 9781003367840 (ebook)
Subjects: LCSH: Mental illness--Philosophy. | Psychiatry--Philosophy. | Philosophy of mind.
Classification: LCC RC437.5 .D46 2024 (print) | LCC RC437.5 (ebook) | DDC 616.89/14--dc23/eng/20230830
LC record available at https://lccn.loc.gov/2023025445
LC ebook record available at https://lccn.loc.gov/2023025446

ISBN: 978-1-032-43546-6 (hbk)
ISBN: 978-1-032-43547-3 (pbk)
ISBN: 978-1-003-36784-0 (ebk)

DOI: 10.4324/9781003367840

Typeset in Sabon
by SPi Technologies India Pvt Ltd (Straive)

For Nives

Contents

Acknowledgments

My first thanks are to Geert Keil and Andreas Heinz for the fruitful discussions, their sharp feedback, and their enduring support. A special thanks goes to my dear friend Romy Jaster for being my extended mind. For helpful conversations, comments, and encouragement, I thank Dorothee Bleisch, Inga Bones, Stefan Brandt, Björn Brodowski, Andreas Cremonini, Alexander Dinges, Gen Eickers, Gerhard Ernst, Simon Gaus, Rebekka Hufendiek, Christian Kietzmann, Martin Klein, Herbert Kley, Muriel Koch, Nora Kreft, Beate Krickel, Jens Kulenkampff, David Lanius, Rosario La Sala, Steffen Lesle, Tamara Lewin, Jennifer Smalligan Marušić, Erasmus Mayr, Nico Scarano, Christoph Schamberger, Stephan Schmid, Sebastian Schmidt, Luz Christopher Seiberth, Thomas Smettan, Henrik Walter, Konstantin Weber, Anna Welpinghus, Hannes Worthmann, Barbara Vetter, and Julia Zakkou. Without all your valuable input and support, I could not have finished this book.

I thank the Deutsche Forschungsgemeinschaft (DFG, German Research Foundation) for the funding I received while working at the "Human Abilities" Centre for Advanced Studies in the Humanities (Grant number 409272951).

I thank my grandmothers Heda and Mara for giving me resilience, my father Zlatko for his unbeatable optimism, and my mother Nives for her unbeatable love. I am deeply grateful to my brother, Berislav Marušić, who is my role model, both as a philosopher and as a person. My deepest gratitude is to Jan Hempelmann and our child Toni Nives for: the good life.

Introduction

Nives was a psychiatrist, born in Croatia in 1952. She migrated to Switzerland with her second husband in 1984 and eventually opened her own psychiatric practice. She had two children: a boy from her first marriage and a girl from her second. Nives had an on-and-off relationship with her second husband. In 1995, he moved to Norway, after which they maintained a long-distance relationship, seeing each other only during holidays. Nives died in 2007 as a result of heart failure.

Nives used psychoactive substances from her 20s until her death, self-medicating with antidepressants and anxiolytics, and, occasionally, with antipsychotics. She often asked her children to get her these self-prescribed drugs from the pharmacy. Over the years, her tolerance for these substances increased. Eventually, she took around 150 pills of lorazepam (Temesta) over the course of a weekend. On New Year's Eve in 1999, she overdosed on these drugs and was hospitalized against her will.

By that time, Nives' day-to-day life was dominated by around 12 to 14 hours of work. When she had spare time, she would be too exhausted to engage in any recreational activities. For the most part, Nives would stay in bed to recover during these periods. Over the years, she lost contact with almost all of her friends and the long-distance relationship with her husband was fraught with many fierce disputes. She cried often and for large parts of the day. She mentioned several times that her children were her only reason for living.

In 1995, Nives was diagnosed with myocarditis. Although her heart condition improved over time, she became ill increasingly more often. She had migraines, frequent infections, and recurrent cystitis, which she self-medicated with antibiotics. Her condition caused her to increasingly miss work. To compensate for her financial losses, she would work extra hours when she was not ill, and to compensate for her overbearing workload, she would spend exorbitant amounts of money on luxury goods. Because of this, she entered a downward spiral of illness, work, and money spending. She died on the day she was meant to file for bankruptcy, which would have been the second time she had had to do this.

DOI: 10.4324/9781003367840-1

On the face of it, Nives did not merely have serious "problems in living," to use a phrase coined by Thomas Szasz (1960); she also appears to
have been suffering from a mental disorder. But what about Nives' mental
condition is it that makes it "disordered"? More generally, we may ask
what it is for any individual to have a mental disorder. Answering this
question is the main focus of this book. My aim is to contribute to a better
understanding of mental disorder by exploring how the concept of mental
disorder relates to other relevant concepts. More specifically, my goal is to
develop a definition of the technical concept associated with the term
"mental disorder" via the method of conceptual explication. I propose that
to explicate that concept we have to refer to abilities, reasons, and harm.
In light of this, I call the resulting view the "Rehability View" (henceforth,
RHA), which is a portmanteau of "REasons," "Harm," and "ABILITY."
I will argue that RHA is preferable to the major competing conceptions of
mental disorder proposed within the contemporary literature on philosophy of psychiatry.

In order to elucidate where conceptual explication lies within a broader
map of methods, it is helpful to distinguish between two types of questions
we might ask concerning the concept of mental disorder:

1 What is (or, what are) our actual mental disorder concept(s)?
2 What should our mental disorder concept(s) be so that it is (or they are)
   useful to us for particular purposes?

To answer the first question, we must engage in *conceptual analysis*. Here,
our aim is to make explicit our actual concepts of thought, or the concepts
that underlie our everyday linguistic practice. To analyze the concept of
mental disorder is to propose a definition that captures our actual (correct)
ascriptions of mental disorder. To answer the second question, we must
engage in *conceptual explication* (henceforth, explication).[1] Here, our aim
is, as Ruth Millikan puts it, to "fashion" a concept "that will do a certain
job" (1984, 2). More specifically, I understand "explication" in Rudolf
Carnap's sense, which is the process of

> making more exact a vague or not quite exact concept used in everyday
> life or in an earlier stage of scientific or logical development, or rather
> of replacing it by a newly constructed, more exact concept.
>
> (1947, 7–8)

Typically, such an explication is "conservative" in the sense that it respects
as many of the core uses of the concept-to-be-explicated as possible, given
the defined purposes, although it need not do so. To explicate the concept
of mental disorder is to propose a definition that fits the purposes for which

we (should) make ascriptions of mental disorder in the first place. I will pursue a conservative explication of the technical concept of mental disorder and shall elaborate on the method of explication (clarifying who "we" are) in Chapter 1.[2]

My project raises two questions: (1) why do we need a definition of the concept of mental disorder at all, and (2) why should we develop such a definition by means of a conservative explication? I propose that we need to define the concept of mental disorder for certain scientific and normative purposes. Broadly, we need it to determine the scope of psychopathology and to help us settle certain normative questions such as (a) whether an individual should seek psychiatric or psychotherapeutic treatment and (b) whether they should be (partly) exempt or excused from certain social, legal, or moral obligations. Furthermore, it is problematic that currently no fixed definition can be satisfyingly given, given that the field of mental disorder is a contested area. There are significant disagreements as to whether certain mental conditions do, or should, fall under the concept of mental disorder. These disagreements need to be settled in a non-arbitrary way (if this is at all possible). I will argue that only the method of explication can help us settle these disagreements because it is only this method that is concerned explicitly with *purposes*. It is precisely in virtue of the purposes for which we use, or should use, the concept of mental disorder that will provide the means to settle the disagreements in question (leaving out the issues of vagueness and borderline cases which is a separate topic). In addition, an explication of the concept of mental disorder should be conservative because we should respect and acknowledge the scientific insights made by relevant disciplines. I will elaborate further on the purposes of the concept of mental disorder in Section 1.2 and defend the method of explication in Section 1.4.

In the remainder of the Introduction, I will (1) make some remarks on terminology, (2) give an overview of the major prevalent views of the concept of mental disorder, and (3) present an outline of the rest of the book.

I.1 Terminology

It is important to distinguish between (a) words or terms, (b) concepts, and (c) properties. Roughly, we *use* words and, by more or less systematically doing so, we succeed to *express* concepts and to *ascribe* properties. To avoid conflating a concept, F, with the property of F or with the meaning of the word "F," I follow the convention of writing the names of concepts in small capitals. For the purposes of my project, we can therefore distinguish between the term "mental disorder," the concept MENTAL DISORDER, and the property of having a mental disorder. To ascribe to an individual, S, a mental disorder (by saying "S has a mental disorder") is to claim that

S has the property of a mental disorder or that their mental condition falls under the concept MENTAL DISORDER.

My project is primarily concerned with concepts. Concepts are categories and the term "concept" can refer to both a category of thought or a category underlying our linguistic practice.[3] There are colloquial concepts, which underlie our everyday linguistic practice, and technical concepts, which underlie our linguistic practice in technical, or scientific, contexts. My project is primarily concerned with technical concepts, most notably, with the concept MENTAL DISORDER that underlies our linguistic practice in clinical psychology and psychiatry.

Concepts may be characterized by their extension and an intension. Generally, a concept's intension refers to the concept's content or definition. Its extension refers to the set of entities to which the definition applies or to which we refer in our actual (correct) use of the term(s) associated with that concept. For example, the intension of the concept BACHELOR is UNMARRIED MAN, and its extension is the set of all men who are unmarried. For something to "fall under a concept," or "into a category," is to be a member of that concept's extension.[4] Any proposed definition of MENTAL DISORDER may be called a "conception" or "view." It is possible to develop a conception by many different methods (analysis, explication, stipulation, or other). I, however, specifically advocate for the use of the method of explication to develop a conception of MENTAL DISORDER.

We sometimes use different terms to express one and the same concept and we may even use one term to express different concepts. For example, the terms "human" and "Mensch," the latter being the German translation of the former, are different terms for the same concept. In the health literature, there is a debate on whether the terms "disease," "illness," and "sickness" also express the same concept (see Hofmann 2002). The term "disease," however, is a case in which one term is used to express at least two different concepts. Taken widely, "disease" may be defined as "every condition of an individual that departs from health." Taken narrowly, "disease" may be defined as "a condition of an individual that departs from health which is not a wound or an injury." These appear to be different concepts, given their difference in intension and extension.

I shall use two umbrella terms for all conditions that depart from health (including diseases, illnesses, disabilities, injuries, wounds, and so on), namely "disorder" and "pathological condition."[5] Accordingly, I shall use "mental disorder" and "pathological mental condition" to refer to all departures from mental health. Likewise, I shall use the terms "bodily disorder" and "pathological bodily condition" for all departures from bodily health.[6] Here, the question may be raised as to why the discussion is not centered around the term "disease," or even "illness." While it seems unintuitive to call wounds such as paper cuts "diseases" or "illnesses," despite the fact that this may be true in some strict sense of the terms, these examples suggest that our colloquial use of "disease" and "illness" express a narrower concept than our technical term, as it does not cover *all* departures from health in its extension. Using "disease" or "illness" as an umbrella term could easily confuse their technical uses with their more colloquial ones. Because I am interested in a technical concept, it is fitting to use an exclusively technical term. Moreover, while my choice is merely terminological, it does not presuppose that MENTAL DISORDER and BODILY DISORDER are best understood as subcategories of a common and more general category DISORDER.

I.2 Prevalent Views[7]

I assume that nobody sincerely denies that the *phenomena* we call "mental disorder" (or that we believe fall under the concept MENTAL DISORDER) exist. Some people experience intense fear in public spaces and rarely leave their houses. It seems uncontroversial that such cases exist. However, what *is* controversial is whether the set or class of phenomena we call "mental disorder," which is determined by its extension, also constitutes a unified concept or category of MENTAL DISORDER.[8] In other words, it might be contested whether there is a unified intension, that is, a coherent set of conditions for membership: conditions that all the members of the class of phenomena we call "mental disorder", and only those members, fulfill.

Some authors argue that it is not possible to give a meaningful definition of "mental disorder" because the term itself is an oxymoron. Szasz (1960, 1961), for instance, claims that mental disorder is a "myth" and could be interpreted along these lines.[9] Derek Bolton (2008) and Bengt Brülde (2010) argue that there is no single (or no stable), concept MENTAL DISORDER, but that there are a couple of different, but similar, ones. As such, we may label them MENTAL DISORDER$_1$, MENTAL DISORDER$_2$, and MENTAL DISORDER$_3$, etc. On their view, there is no single definition of MENTAL DISORDER that can fulfill all desiderata necessary for a comprehensive view of mental disorder.[10]

Some authors merely deny that a definition of MENTAL DISORDER in terms of necessary and sufficient conditions can be given (see Lilienfeld and Marino 1995, Mackinejad and Sharifi 2006, Hucklenbroich 2008, Keil and Stoecker 2017, and Walker and Rogers 2018). Instead, they argue for a definition of a different type; some authors argue in favor of a definition in terms of similarity to a prototype akin to Wittgenstein's idea of "family resemblance." To take a specific example, Geert Keil and Ralf Stoecker (2017) argue that MENTAL DISORDER is a so-called cluster concept. They take a cluster concept to be explicitly or implicitly defined on the basis of an open or closed list of criteria, such that none of these criteria and no combination thereof are both necessary and jointly sufficient for the phenomenon's falling under that concept.

(2017, 56–57)

Because I am interested in an explication of the concept MENTAL DISORDER in terms of necessary and sufficient conditions, I treat skepticism about whether the concept can be defined as a last resort. It remains to be seen whether a project of the kind I pursue will turn out to be successful. Regardless of any skeptical concerns we may have, aiming for a comprehensive and unified explication may nevertheless give us important insights into the phenomena of mental disorder, even if, ultimately, we do not succeed in reaching a consensus.

Furthermore, despite the skeptical concern noted earlier, there are already many influential conceptions of what it is to have a mental disorder. It is difficult to systematize them, given that the views have both significant differences and overlap. In order to group the main positions insightfully and comprehensibly, I propose to cluster the major prevalent conceptions of MENTAL DISORDER around the aspect they most heavily focus on. These are the aspects of (1) harm, (2) action, and (3) biological function. Though not all authors take themselves to pursue an explication, I shall treat their views—for methodical reasons—as if they do. As my project is to explicate MENTAL DISORDER, any conception that "does the job" may be considered satisfying even if it was not originally proposed as an explication, but, rather, as a conceptual analysis.

First, I shall refer to conceptions that focus on HARM (without referring to biological functions) as "Harm Views" (see, for example, Clouser, Culver, and Gert 1981, Reznek 1991, Cooper 2007). Proponents of Harm Views hold that, for an individual to have a mental disorder, it is necessary that they be in a harmful mental condition. Most Harm Views are actually Harm⁺ Views because simply being in a harmful mental condition is clearly not sufficient for having a mental disorder. An individual who experiences grief, for example, may be in a harmful mental condition, but they may not have a mental disorder.

Second, I shall refer to conceptions that focus on ACTION as "Action Views." Proponents of Action Views hold that, for an individual to have a mental disorder, it is necessary that the individual fails to φ, or does not have a certain ability to φ, where φ is an action. I focus on two views in particular: Bill Fulford's (1989) view, which claims that mental disorders necessarily involve a failure of ordinary action, and Lennart Nordenfelt's (1995, 2001, 2007) view, which claims that mental disorder necessarily involves a failure to achieve the goals necessary for one's "minimal happiness."[11]

Third, I shall refer to conceptions that focus on BIOLOGICAL FUNCTION as "Biological Function Views." Proponents of Biological Function Views hold that, for an individual to have a mental disorder, it is necessary (and on one version, sufficient) that an individual be in a condition that results from a failure of some mental mechanism to perform at least one of its biological functions.[12] Biological Function Views are the most comprehensively developed and influential conceptions of DISORDER, the two most significant versions being Christopher Boorse's (1975, 1976a, 1976b, 1977, 1997, 2002, 2014) "Biostatistical Theory" (BST) and Jerome Wakefield's (1992a, 1992b, 1999, 2006) "Harmful Dysfunction Analysis" (HDA).[13] Boorse develops his conception by considering cases of bodily disorder, claiming that his BST applies to cases of mental disorder as well. Wakefield's conception, however, is developed in specific application to cases of mental disorder. Contrary to Boorse, Wakefield argues that the presence of a biological dysfunction is not sufficient for the presence of a disorder, as, according to him, it is also necessary that the individual be harmed.

In addition to the aforementioned views, there are sketches of views that focus on the aspects of INTENTIONALITY, RATIONALITY, or REASONS (see Edwards 1981, Bolton 2001, Graham 2010). Given that my view builds on and specifies what I take to be the gist of these views, I will not discuss them separately but refer to them in Chapter 4.

Before moving on, I shall make three general points about the literature on MENTAL DISORDER and BODILY DISORDER to orientate my project among them.

First, BODILY DISORDER is often the primary focus in this literature, which is justified through the assumption that we already have a firm grasp of our use of the term "bodily disorder" (or "disease"). Authors imply that, if we have an adequate analysis or explication of BODILY DISORDER, we will also have an adequate analysis or explication of MENTAL DISORDER. To put it differently, we may apply the concept DISORDER, as it appears in BODILY DISORDER, appropriately to the realm of the mental (see Fulford 1989, 2018, Fulford, Thornton, and Graham 2006).[14] On this view, MENTAL DISORDER and BODILY DISORDER are subcategories of the more general category DISORDER.

Second, the literature on mental disorder appears to focus more on the concept DISORDER (or the disorder/non-disorder distinction) than on the concept MENTAL (or the bodily/mental distinction). If the latter concept is discussed at all, it is often in reference to the metaphysical mind/body problem. It is rarely discussed what is *mental* about mental disorder, that is, in what sense a mental disorder is "mental."[15]

In this book, I attempt to explicate MENTAL DISORDER in terms of clear cases of mental disorder. Furthermore, I will argue that, in order to account for what is mental about mental disorder, we have to take an individual's reasons-responsiveness into account. While deriving a conception of MENTAL DISORDER *via* an analysis of BODILY DISORDER is theoretically elegant because it allows us to develop a unified theory of both mental and bodily disorders, it is also somewhat stipulated and potentially highly revisionary. The fact that we can use the term "disorder" to refer to either mental or bodily cases of disorder does not provide us with sufficient reason to believe that these terms should be conceived of as subcategories of a more general category DISORDER. Whether or not mental and bodily disorder fall under said category should be treated as an open question and not taken for granted.

My project, however, will not be concerned with the metaphysical mind/body problem. Rather, I follow Dominic Murphy (2006, 9) in assuming an "unsophisticated materialism"; mental states, events, or processes are "rooted" in bodily states, events, or processes. Mental phenomena, in other words, can be said to be token-identical (but not necessarily type-identical), to supervene on, or to be realized by bodily phenomena. With the exception of eliminative materialism, my conceptual project should not be undermined by any of the alternative metaphysical positions concerning the mind/body problem (though it may raise doubt as to whether type-identity views are plausible). However, if eliminative materialism is true, then any conception of MENTAL DISORDER is in trouble anyway.

Third, a large part of the literature on the concept MENTAL DISORDER is concerned with whether the concept can be analyzed in purely naturalistic terms or whether normative elements or values are essential to it.[16] Proponents of the former view can be called "naturalists," while proponents of the latter view are referred to as "normativists" (or "value theorists"). Harm Views and Action Views are typically normativist views, while Biological Function Views are typically naturalist. This debate is occasionally framed in terms of the dichotomies "objectivism versus subjectivism/constructivism" or "facts versus values" (see Fulford 1989, 2018, Murphy 2006). However, it is misleading to frame the debate in these terms because it assumes that normative claims cannot be objectively true or that there cannot be facts about what is valuable. Given the extensive work undertaken on this subject, I shall not make the same assumptions going forward.

It is necessary to clarify on what claim naturalists and normativists disagree. Typically, the naturalist holds that, for an individual to have a mental disorder, it is necessary that they be in a condition which is either caused or constituted by a mechanism not performing its biological function. Normativists, however, hold that for an individual to have a mental disorder, it is necessary that they be in a bad condition, or in a condition in which they, in some sense, "should not be" or "are not supposed to be in." In principle, these claims are not incompatible, and it is possible to simultaneously endorse both (see Wakefield 1992a). While naturalists typically reject that for an individual to have a mental disorder, it is *necessary* for them to be in a bad condition or a condition in which they "should not be," they would nevertheless concede that having a mental disorder *usually, statistically normally, typically* or *often* comes with being in bad condition. According to naturalists, it is consistent to state "S has a mental disorder, but S is not in a bad condition." This, however, is precisely what normativists reject, as they claim that to have a mental disorder *just is* to say that an individual is in a bad mental condition or that their mental condition is in some sense "not as it is supposed to be."[17]

In addition, the naturalist typically claims that, while ascriptions of mental disorder and ascriptions of bad conditions often correlate, it is a contingent fact that they do so. This correlation may be explained by the fact that we contingently value conditions of mental health, and if we did not value those conditions as we do, or if they were not as valuable to us as they are, having a mental disorder would not be considered a bad thing. Nevertheless, according to the naturalist, it might still be possible to ascribe mental disorders in a coherent way.

Should we accept naturalism or normativism? This depends, in part, on which method one pursues. If one is committed to a conceptual analysis of MENTAL DISORDER, then one would have to wait until the analysis is complete before concluding which position one should accept. In contrast, if one employs the method of explication, then answering whether we should accept naturalism or normativism depends, in part, on the purposes for which one wants to explicate MENTAL DISORDER. One goal of my project is to explicate that concept for certain practical or normative purposes (see Section 1.2); therefore normative, or evaluative, aspects are likely to appear within my explication. However, given my interest in an explication for theoretical or scientific purposes, the explication that follows should at least make room for naturalistic concepts such as BIOLOGICAL FUNCTION.

I.3 Outline

I conclude this Introduction by giving an outline of the rest of the book.

Chapter 1: The Method describes and defends the method of *explication* for the technical concept MENTAL DISORDER. I describe this method in contrast to *conceptual analysis*. Furthermore, I propose and elaborate on a set of scientific and normative purposes for which the concept MENTAL DISORDER should be used. This is (1) to determine the scope of psychopathology and (2) to help us settle (a) who is entitled to psychiatric or psychotherapeutic treatment and (b) who can be (partly) exempt or excused from certain social, legal, or moral obligations. The chapter also delineates the actual technical usage of the concept in question and proposes four adequacy conditions for any comprehensive explication of

MENTAL DISORDER for the aforementioned purposes. Lastly, I defend the proposed method against some potential objections.

Chapter 2: Harm Views and Action Views describes the major prevalent Harm Views and Action Views of mental disorder (except for those that refer also to biological dysfunctions) and evaluates them in light of the adequacy conditions outlined in Chapter 1. I argue that the presented Harm Views and Action Views do not provide a satisfactory explication of MENTAL DISORDER given the scientific and normative purposes we should use it for. Nonetheless, I propose that harm is a promising candidate for capturing at least some aspects which are relevant for the concept's normative purposes.

Chapter 3: Biological Function Views describes the major prevalent Biological Function Views of mental disorder and evaluates them in light of the adequacy conditions outlined in Chapter 1. I argue that Biological Function Views do not provide a satisfactory explication of MENTAL DISORDER given the scientific and normative purposes we should use it for. Nonetheless, I propose that any satisfactory explication of MENTAL DISORDER should be compatible with the claim that at least some mental disorders can be explained by reference to biological dysfunctions.

Chapter 4: The Rehability View presents and motivates the view I want to defend. On RHA, having a mental disorder is a matter of (1) being *unable* to respond adequately to some of one's available (apparent) *reasons* for (or against) some of one's reasons-sensitive attitudes or actions and (2) being *harmed* by the condition underlying or resulting from that inability. In the course of this chapter, I elaborate extensively on the concepts ABILITY, REASONS, and HARM. Furthermore, I develop and illustrate RHA by way of a case study of anxiety disorder.

Chapter 5: Defending the Rehability View argues that we should accept RHA for the following three reasons. First, RHA meets all of the adequacy conditions from Chapter 1 to a high degree. RHA captures (1) the distinction between mental health and mental disorder, (2) the distinction between mental disorder and bodily disorder, and (3) the distinction between mental disorder and deviances from social, legal, or moral norms. In addition, it (4) clarifies what it is about having a mental disorder that helps us settle certain normative questions such as (a) who is entitled to psychiatric or psychotherapeutic treatment and (b) who can be (partly) exempt or excused from certain social, legal, or moral obligations. Second, RHA avoids the problems faced by the views discussed in Chapters 2 and 3. Third, RHA can be defended against some potential objections, objections that question the relevance of reasons-sensitivity and harm when it comes to mental disorder.

Chapter 6: Case Study: Addictive Disorder presents a definition of "addictive disorder" in terms of RHA. This definition refers to the concepts of desire, inability, harm, tolerance, and withdrawal. The main focus of the chapter is the concept ABILITY. I argue that RHA can capture and clarify (1) the distinction between disorder and non-disorder and (2) the distinction between addictive disorder and other similar types of mental disorders (such as obsessive-compulsive disorder). Furthermore, I argue that a competing view put forward by Walter Sinnott-Armstrong and Hanna Pickard (2013) has trouble capturing these distinctions. The aim of this chapter is then twofold: to illustrate RHA with an example (addictive disorder) and to employ that example in demonstrating RHA's fruitfulness.

The *Conclusion* summarizes RHA and emphasizes a few things that the view does not imply. RHA implies neither (a) that an individual with a mental disorder is completely or globally irrational, nor (b) that their life is, all things considered, not "good enough," nor (c) that they cannot overcome their mental disorder (on their own). Furthermore, two conclusions are drawn. First, RHA suggests that debates about whether those who have a mental disorder, "can" or "cannot" do otherwise are futile. Second, RHA suggests that psychiatric treatment and psychotherapy could be about (1) *enabling* individuals with mental disorders to cope with their "problems in living" and/or (2) relieving the *harm* they are subjected to by their inability.

Notes

1 See Daly (2010) for an introduction to different philosophical methods and Cappelen (2018) for a discussion of "conceptual engineering" more generally.
2 Occasionally, the term "conceptual explication" is used to label, what I call, "conceptual analysis" and *vice versa*. My project is not to argue for a certain definition of these terms, and therefore I do not insist on my use of terminology. Furthermore, there may be other conceptual projects that do not fit neatly into this distinction, such as the "Canberra plan" by Lewis (1994) and Jackson (1998). In addition, I do not claim that this set of philosophical methods is an exhaustive list. I merely use the distinction to introduce my method. For similar approaches with regard to the concept DISEASE, see Schwartz (2007, 2014), and Griffiths and Matthewson (2018).
3 See Margolis and Laurence (1999) for different theories of concepts.
4 I shall use the expression "to use a concept F" as a loose way of stating "to state that something falls (or does not fall) under the concept F."
5 I choose these terms to demarcate the areas of discussion for lack of a better linguistic taxonomy to do so. This is because, when discussing mental disorder, problems arise in terms of negative implicit connotations and implicatures associated with particular terms. If we use a certain term with a degrading attitude, the term itself acquires a connotation that involves the degradation of the phenomena to which we refer by using that term. To remove the connotation, we may start to use another term to denote the same type of phenomena. But this does not preclude the fact that the new term may be used with the same degrading attitude. I do not intend to use the terms "mental disorder" and "pathological mental condition" with a degrading attitude, but if any reader

finds them inappropriate, they may substitute them with any other term they find more suitable.

6 In the literature, various umbrella terms are used, for instance "disease" (Boorse 1975, 1977, Cooper 2002), "malady" (Clouser, Culver, and Gert 1981), and "pathological condition" (Boorse 1997, 2014).

7 Since my project is concerned with the question of "demarcation" or with "evaluative sorting" (Ross 2005, 127), the following overview is restricted to the prevalent views of the concept MENTAL DISORDER that are relevant to that end.

8 A concept or category always creates a corresponding class, but, perhaps, not *vice versa.*

9 For different interpretations of Szasz' main claim, see Reznek (1991, chapter 5).

10 Brown (1985), Hesslow (1993), Kincaid (2008), Vickers, Basch, and Kattan (2008), and Ereshefsky (2009) go even further to argue that we do not need, or we should even give up, seeking a definition of DISEASE (in my terminology: DISORDER).

11 The predecessors of Nordenfelt's view are Whitbeck (1978, 1981) and Pörn (1984). Another ability-based view can be found in Gaete (2008).

12 It is worth noting that the definition of "mental disorder" in the fifth edition of the *Diagnostic and Statistical Manual of Mental Disorders (DSM-5)* also refers to dysfunctions and harm:

> A mental disorder is a syndrome characterized by clinically significant disturbance in an individual's cognition, emotion regulation, or behavior that reflects a dysfunction in the psychological, biological, or developmental processes underlying mental functioning. Mental disorders are usually associated with significant distress or disability in social, occupational, or other important activities. An expectable or culturally approved response to a common stressor or loss, such as the death of a loved one, is not a mental disorder. Socially deviant behavior (e.g., political, religious, or sexual) and conflicts that are primarily between the individual and society are not mental disorders unless the deviance or conflict results from a dysfunction in the individual, as described above.
>
> (APA 2013, 20)

This definition is informative, but it is not sufficiently clear. It raises several questions. For instance, what is a "disturbance," and what exactly does it mean to have a "clinically significant" disturbance? What are "dysfunctions," and how do psychological, biological, and developmental processes relate to one another? What does it mean for them to be "reflected" in a clinically significant disturbance and to "underlie" mental functioning? It appears that more theoretical work needs be done to clarify this working definition.

13 Papineau (1994), Schramme (2010), and Heinz (2014, 2017, 2018) have similar views.

14 See also Szasz (1960, 1961) and Kendell (1975) who define DISORDER with respect to cases of bodily disorder and come to different conclusions about whether anything falls under it.

15 Exceptions are Bolton and Hill (1998), Arpaly (2005), Brülde and Radovic (2006), and Wakefield (2006).

16 See Engelhardt (1975), Reznek (1987), Fulford (1989, 2018), Nordenfelt (1995, 2001, 2007), and Cooper (2002) for normativist views. See Boorse (1975, 1977, 1997, 2014), Murphy (2006), Ananth (2008), De Block (2008), and Schramme (2010) for naturalist views. Wakefield (1992a) proposes both a

normativist and a naturalist view. See Thornton (2007) and Kingma (2014) for a helpful discussion of this distinction and Gagné-Julien (2020) for an attempt to overcome this dichotomy.

17 Fulford (1989, 2018) that naturalists such as Boorse *define* "disorder" (and similar terms) in non-evaluative terms but are not able to *use* them in a non-evaluative way.

References

American Psychiatric Association (APA). 2013. *Diagnostic and Statistical Manual of Mental Disorders: DSM-5*. Arlington: American Psychiatric Association.

Ananth, Mahesh. 2008. *In Defense of an Evolutionary Concept of Health*. Aldershot: Ashgate.

Arpaly, Nomy. 2005. "How It Is Not 'Just Like Diabetes': Mental Disorders and the Moral Psychologist." *Philosophical Issues* 15 (1): 282–298.

Bolton, Derek. 2001. "Problems in the Definition of 'Mental disorder'." *The Philosophical Quarterly* 51 (203): 182–199.

———. 2008. *What Is Mental Disorder? An Essay in Philosophy, Science, and Values*. Oxford: Oxford University Press.

Bolton, Derek, and Jonathan Hill. 1998. *Mind, Meaning and Mental Disorder*. Oxford: Oxford University Press.

Boorse, Christopher. 1975. "On the Distinction between Disease and Illness." *Philosophy and Public Affairs* 5 (1): 49–68.

———. 1976a. "What a Theory of Mental Health Should Be." *Journal for the Theory of Social Behaviour* 6 (1): 61–84.

———. 1976b. "Wright on Functions." *Philosophical Review* 85 (1): 70–86.

———. 1977. "Health as a Theoretical Concept." *Philosophy of Science* 44 (4): 542–573.

———. 1997. "A Rebuttal on Health." In *What Is Disease?*, edited by James M. Humber and Robert F. Almeder, 1–134. New Jersey: Humana Press.

———. 2002. "A Rebuttal on Functions." In *Functions: New Essays in the Philosophy of Psychology and Biology*, edited by André Ariew, Robert C. Cummins, and Mark Perlman, 63–112. Oxford: Oxford University Press.

———. 2014. "A Second Rebuttal on Health." *Journal of Medicine and Philosophy* 39 (6): 683–724.

Brown, W. Miller. 1985. "On Defining 'Disease'." *The Journal of Medicine and Philosophy* 10: 311–328.

Brülde, Bengt. 2010. "On Defining 'Mental Disorder': Purposes and Conditions of Adequacy." *Theoretical Medicine and Bioethics* 31 (1): 19–33.

Brülde, Bengt, and Filip Radovic. 2006. "What Is Mental About Mental Disorder?" *Philosophy, Psychiatry, and Psychology* 13 (2): 99–116.

Cappelen, Herman. 2018. *Fixing Language: An Essay on Conceptual Engineering*. Oxford: Oxford University Press.

Carnap, Rudolf. 1947. *Meaning and Necessity*. Chicago: University of Chicago Press.

Clouser, K. Danner, Charles M. Culver, and Bernard Gert. 1981. "Malady: A New Treatment of Disease." *The Hastings Center Report* 11 (3): 29–37.

Cooper, Rachel. 2002. "Disease." *Studies in History and Philosophy of Science* 33 (2): 263–282.

———. 2007. *Psychiatry and Philosophy of Science*. Durham: Acumen.

Daly, Chris. 2010. *An Introduction to Philosophical Methods*. Toronto: Broadview Press.

De Block, Andreas. 2008. "Why Mental Disorders Are Just Mental Dysfunctions (and Nothing More): Some Darwinian Arguments." *Studies in History and Philosophy of Biological and Biomedical Sciences* 39: 338–346.

Edwards, Rem B. 1981. "Mental Health as Rational Autonomy." *Journal of Medicine and Philosophy* 6 (3): 309–322.

Engelhardt, H. Tristram Jr. 1975. "The Concepts of Health and Disease." In *Evaluation and Explanation in the Biomedical Sciences*, edited by H. Tristram Engelhardt Jr., and Stuart F. Spicker (1st edn), 125–141. Dordrecht: D. Reidel Publishing Company.

Ereshefsky, Marc. 2009. "Defining 'Health' and 'Disease'." *Studies in History and Philosophy of Science* 40 (3): 221–227.

Fulford, William K. M. 1989. *Moral Theory and Medical Practice*. Cambridge: Cambridge University Press.

———. 2018. "Was ist eine Psychische Störung? Die Philosophie der normalen Sprache als Ausgangspunkt." *Deutsche Zeitschrift für Philosophie* 66 (2): 205–227.

Fulford, William K. M., Tim Thornton, and George Graham, eds. 2006. *Oxford Textbook of Philosophy and Psychiatry*. Oxford: Oxford University Press.

Gaete, Alfredo. 2008. "The Concept of Mental Disorder: A Proposal." *Philosophy, Psychiatry, and Psychology* 15 (4): 327–339.

Gagné-Julien, Anne-Marie. 2020. "Towards a Socially Constructed and Objective Concept of Mental Disorder." *Synthese* 198 (10): 9401–9426.

Graham, George. 2010. *The Disordered Mind: An Introduction to Philosophy of Mind and Mental Illness*. London: Routledge.

Griffiths, Paul E., and John Matthewson. 2018. "Evolution, Dysfunction, and Disease: A Reappraisal." *British Journal for Philosophy of Science* 69: 301–327.

Heinz, Andreas. 2014. *Der Begriff der psychischen Krankheit*. Berlin: Suhrkamp.

———. 2017. *A New Understanding of Mental Disorders: Computational Models for Dimensional Psychiatry*. Cambridge, MA: MIT Press.

———. 2018. "Geistlose Hirne und hirnlose Geister: Zum Umgang mit dem Begriff psychischer Krankheit." *Deutsche Zeitschrift für Philosophie* 66 (2): 228–242.

Hesslow, Germund. 1993. "Do We Need a Concept of Disease?" *Theoretical Medicine and Bioethics* 14 (1): 1–14.

Hofmann, Bjørn. 2002. "On the Triad Disease, Illness and Sickness." *Medicine and Philosophy* 27 (6): 651–673.

Hucklenbroich, Peter. 2008. "'Normal – Anders – Krank': Begriffsklärungen und theoretische Grundlagen zum Krankheitsbegriff." In *Normal – Anders – Krank? Akzeptanz, Stigmatisierung und Pathologisierung im Kontext der Medizin*, edited by Dominik Groß, Sabine Müller, and Jan Steinmetzer, 3–31. Berlin: Medizinisch Wissenschaftliche Verlagsgesellschaft.

Jackson, Frank. 1998. *From Metaphysics to Ethics: A Defense of Conceptual Analysis*. Oxford: Oxford University Press.

Keil, Geert, and Ralf Stoecker. 2017. "Disease as a Vague and Thick Cluster Concept." In *Vagueness in Psychiatry*, edited by Geert Keil, Lara Keuck, and Rico Hauswald, 46–75. Oxford: Oxford University Press.

Kendell, Robert E. 1975. "The Concept of Disease and Its Implications for Psychiatry." *The British Journal of Psychiatry* 127 (4): 305–315.

Kincaid, Harold. 2008. "Do We Need Theory to Study Disease?" *Perspectives in Biology and Medicine* 51: 367–378.

Kingma, Elselijn. 2014. "Naturalism About Health and Disease: Adding Nuance for Progress." *Journal of Medicine and Philosophy* 39 (6): 590–608.

Lewis, David. 1994. "Reduction of Mind." In *Companion to the Philosophy of Mind*, edited by Samuel Guttenplan, 412–431. Oxford: Blackwell.

Lilienfeld, Scott O., and Lori Marino. 1995. "Mental Disorder as a Roschian Concept: A Critique of Wakefield's 'Harmful Dysfunction' Analysis." *Journal of Abnormal Psychology* 104 (3): 411–420.

Mackinejad, Kioumars, and Vandad Sharifi. 2006. "Wittgenstein's Philosophy and a Dimensional Approach to the Classification of Mental Disorders: A Preliminary Scheme." *Psychopathology* 39 (3): 126–129.

Margolis, Eric, and Stephen Laurence, eds. 1999. *Concepts. Core Readings*. Cambridge, MA: MIT Press.

Millikan, Ruth G. 1984. *Language, Thought and Other Biological Categories: New Foundations for Realism*. Cambridge, MA: MIT Press.

Murphy, Dominic. 2006. *Psychiatry in the Scientific Image*. Cambridge, MA: MIT Press.

Nordenfelt, Lennart. 1995. *On the Nature of Health an Action-Theoretic Approach* (2nd edn). Dordrecht: Springer.

———. 2001. *Health, Science, and Ordinary Language*. New York: Rodopi.

———. 2007. "The Concepts of Health and Illness Revisited." *Medicine, Health Care and Philosophy* 10 (1): 5–10.

Papineau, David. 1994. "Mental Disorder, Illness, and Biological Disfunction." *Royal Institute of Philosophy Supplements* 37: 73–82.

Pörn, Ingmar. 1984. "An Equilibrium Model of Health." In *Health, Disease, and Causal Explanations in Medicine*, edited by Lennart Nordenfelt and B. Ingemar B. Lindahl, 3–9. Dordrecht: D. Reidel Publishing Company.

Reznek, Lawrie. 1987. *The Nature of Disease*. London: Routledge.

———. 1991. *The Philosophical Defence of Psychiatry*. Florence: Taylor and Francis/Routledge.

Ross, Patricia A. 2005. "Sorting Out the Concept Disorder." *Theoretical Medicine and Bioethics* 26: 115–140.

Schramme, Thomas. 2010. "Can We Define Mental Disorder by Using the Criterion of Mental Dysfunction?" *Theoretical Medicine and Bioethics* 31 (1): 35–47.

Schwartz, Peter H. 2007. "Progress in Defining Disease: Improved Approaches and Increased Impact." *Journal of Medicine and Philosophy* 42: 485–502.

———. 2014. "Reframing the Disease Debate and Defending the Biostatistical Theory." *Journal of Medicine and Philosophy* 39: 572–589.

Sinnott-Armstrong, Walter, and Hanna Pickard. 2013. "What Is Addiction?" In *The Oxford Handbook of Philosophy of Psychiatry*, edited by William K. M.

Fulford, Martin Davies, Richard Gipps, George Graham, John Sadler, Giovanni Stanghellini, and Tim Thornton, 851–865. Oxford: Oxford University Press.

Szasz, Thomas S. 1960. "The Myth of Mental Illness." *American Psychologist* 15: 113–118.

———. 1961. *The Myth of Mental Illness: Foundations of a Theory of Personal Conduct*. New York: Hoeber-Harper.

Thornton, Tim. 2007. *Essential Philosophy of Psychiatry*. Oxford: Oxford University Press.

Vickers, Andrew J., Ethan Basch, and Michael W. Kattan. 2008. "Against Diagnosis." *Annals of Internal Medicine* 149: 200–203.

Wakefield, Jerome C. 1992a. "The Concept of Mental Disorder. On the Boundary between Biological Facts and Social Values." *American Psychologist* 47 (3): 373–388.

———. 1992b. "Disorder as Harmful Dysfunction: A Conceptual Critique of DSM-III-R's Definition of Mental Disorder." *Psychological Review* 99 (2): 232–247.

———. 1999. "Evolutionary versus Prototype Analyses of the Concept of Disorder." *Journal of Abnormal Psychology* 108: 374–399.

———. 2006. "What Makes a Mental Disorder Mental?" *Philosophy, Psychiatry, and Psychology* 13 (2): 123–131.

Walker, Mary J., and Wendy A. Rogers. 2018. "A New Approach to Defining Disease." *Journal of Medicine and Philosophy* 43: 402–420.

Whitbeck, Caroline. 1978. "Four Basic Concepts of Medical Science." In *PSA 1978*, edited by Peter D. Asquith and Ian Hacking, 210–222. East Lansing: Philosophy of Science Association.

———. 1981. "A Theory of Health." In *Concepts of Health and Disease*, edited by Arthur L. Caplan, H. Tristram Engelhardt Jr., and James J. McCartney, 611–626. Reading: Addison-Wesley Publishing Company.

1 The Method

My goal in this book is to develop a definition of MENTAL DISORDER through the method of explication. This chapter describes and defends this method. In Section 1.1, I describe explication in its relation to conceptual analysis. In Section 1.2, I propose a set of purposes for which the concept of MENTAL DISORDER should be used. This section delineates further the concept's actual technical usage. In Section 1.3, I propose four adequacy conditions to be met by any comprehensive explication of MENTAL DISORDER for the purposes outlined in Section 1.2. In Section 1.4, I defend the method of explication for MENTAL DISORDER against some potential objections.

1.1 What Is Explication?

I take "conceptual analysis" to be the project of making explicit the concepts of thought, or the concepts that underlie our actual (colloquial or technical) linguistic practice. Such an analysis is a descriptive endeavor that involves identifying the "deep structure" of our actual thought or linguistic practices.[1] In contrast, "explication" is the project of "fashioning" a concept "that will do a certain job," as Millikan (1984, 2) says. I take the method of explication to be a revisionary project in which we replace an imprecise concept with a more precise one.[2] An explication is "conservative" if it attempts to preserve as much of our actual usage as possible.

On a prevalent view, to *analyze* a concept, F, is to find the (individually) necessary and (jointly) sufficient conditions for something to fall under F (or for the correct ascriptions of F).

Necessary and sufficient conditions are typically defined as follows:

NC A necessary condition for some state of affairs, F, to obtain is a condition that has to be satisfied in order for F to obtain.

SC A sufficient condition for some state of affairs, F, to obtain is a condition that, if satisfied, guarantees that F obtains.

DOI: 10.4324/9781003367840-2

Applied to my project, a necessary condition for an individual, S, to have a mental disorder is a condition that has to be satisfied in order for S to have a mental disorder. A sufficient condition for an individual S to have a mental disorder is a condition that, if satisfied, guarantees that S has a mental disorder.

Importantly, we may draw connections between knowledge of the necessary and sufficient conditions for the correct ascriptions of mental disorder and knowledge about what it is to have a mental disorder. To elaborate, one can distinguish between *metalinguistic statements*, which are about ascriptions of mental disorder, and *object statements*, which are about the phenomena we call "mental disorders." For instance, "The statement 'Nives has a mental disorder' is false" is a metalinguistic statement regarding whether or not the term mental disorder was correctly ascribed. However, the sentence "Nives does not have a mental disorder" is an object statement, that is, a statement about some phenomena in the world. If I know that the sentence "Nives has a mental disorder" is true, then I know that, in actuality, Nives has a mental disorder (and *vice versa*). Therefore, if I know the necessary and sufficient conditions for the correct ascriptions of mental disorder, then I know what it is for some individual to have a mental disorder.

Arguing over analyses makes sense only if they are testable against a backdrop of certain beliefs regarding which entities fall under the concept-to-be-analyzed (the analysandum). Our beliefs may vary, however, in asserting that certain entities (a) clearly do, (b) clearly do not, or (c) neither clearly do nor clearly do not fall under the concept in question. These beliefs will be pre-theoretical if we are analyzing a colloquial concept, but if we are analyzing a technical concept, the relevant beliefs for testing our analysis will be those that are shared by the respective scientific community in which the concept is used and embedded.[3] The result of our analysis (the analysans) needs to pick out the same extensional set as the analysandum. A lack of fit with actual usage is an objection to the analysis. For example, an analysis of our actual technical concept of MENTAL DISORDER cannot imply that schizophrenia is not a mental disorder nor that fear in general is a mental disorder. An analysis is "correct" or "incorrect" depending on whether it captures our actual use of the analysandum, and our technical use of the term "mental disorder" is meant to pick out cases like schizophrenia and not cases like ordinary fear.

The method of *explication*, classically understood, is described by Carnap in the following passage:

> The task of *explication* consists in transforming a given more or less inexact concept into an exact one or, rather, in replacing the first by the second. We call the given concept (or the term used for it) the *explicandum*, and

the exact concept proposed to take the place of the first (or the term proposed for it) the *explicatum*. The explicandum may belong to everyday language or to a previous stage in the development of scientific language.

(1950, 3)

In contrast to conceptual analysis, explication involves a stipulative element. This means that when explicating a concept, we do not aim for a perfect fit between the analysis and actual usage but allow for certain changes. Explication allows us to respect some existing core uses of a concept, or the term(s) associated with it, while being stipulative on others.[4] This has the important consequence that, strictly speaking, an explication cannot be "correct" or "incorrect."

However, an explication may be more or less adequate regarding the *purposes* for which it is made. Carnap suggests the following four conditions to test the adequacy of an explicatum for a given explicandum:

1 The explicatum is to be *similar* to the explicandum in such a way that, in most cases in which the explicandum has so far been used, the explicatum can be used; however, close similarity is not required, and considerable differences are permitted.
2 The characterization of the explicatum, that is, the rules of its use (for instance, in the form of a definition), is to be given in an *exact* form, so as to introduce the explicatum into a well-connected system of scientific concepts.
3 The explicatum is to be a *fruitful* concept, that is, useful for the formulation of many universal statements (empirical laws in the case of a nonlogical concept, logical theorems in the case of a logical concept).
4 The explicatum should be as *simple* as possible; this means, as simple as the more important requirements (1, 2, 3) permit.

(1950, 7)

In essence, an explication can be more or less adequate given how useful it is for certain purposes. To develop an explication, we may start with a concept we already use and, if necessary, we may change our current concept so that the resulting one meets the purposes the concept-to-be-explicated is supposed to serve. Our new concept should be as simple and exact as possible, but it need not be as similar to our current concept as possible.

Following Carnap's view, I propose that to explicate the technical concept MENTAL DISORDER is to formulate a concept that is useful to the relevant scientific and therapeutic communities for certain purposes. The aim of this process is to formulate a set of (individually) necessary and (jointly)

sufficient conditions for an individual to have a mental disorder. The explication should begin with the technical concept MENTAL DISORDER as it is
already used in psychiatry and clinical psychology (but this is, in principle,
open to revision). It should be conservative—that is, aim to preserve as
much of the actual technical usage of MENTAL DISORDER as possible, given
the defined purposes—in order to acknowledge important scientific insights made by relevant disciplines. The new concept should be as simple
and exact as possible.

Before developing an explication, we must first specify the purposes for
which the concept MENTAL DISORDER should be used by the relevant scientific and therapeutic communities, and identify the actual technical usage
that we aim to preserve as much as possible (see Section 1.2). In addition,
we must formulate a set of adequacy conditions to be able to critically
evaluate different explications (see Section 1.3).

1.2 Purposes and Actual Usage

I propose that there are two types of purpose that we should consider in
respect to the use of the concept MENTAL DISORDER: (1) *theoretical or scientific* purposes, and (2) *practical or normative* purposes.[5] I will elaborate
on them in turn. Following this, I will (3) delineate the actual technical
usage of the concept MENTAL DISORDER.

1.2.1 Theoretical or Scientific Purposes

In the theoretical or scientific context, the concept MENTAL DISORDER is
primarily required for the purpose of classification. As theorists, we aim at
a clear, consistent, and non-arbitrary classification of phenomena, including
those which are the proper subject of scientific disciplines such as clinical
psychology or psychiatry. A definition of MENTAL DISORDER enables us to
determine the scope of psychopathology and aids in, as Germund Hesslow
puts it, "organizing a certain body of knowledge" (1993, 4). Furthermore,
a definition helps us to delineate different types of mental disorders in a
systematic and consistent way. With this, we are able to grasp seemingly
disparate types of phenomena as a unified set by making intelligible why
different phenomena fall under the same heading of "mental disorder."

In addition, the concept MENTAL DISORDER is integral to scientific research. A clear, consistent, and non-arbitrary classification enables scientists to conduct proper research on the phenomena in question. Scientists
want to know how the minds of individuals with a mental disorder of a
certain type work relative to the minds of individuals without such a
mental disorder. Following this, scientists compare the incidence and prev-
alence rates of different types of mental disorders, as well as the outcomes

of different therapeutic interventions. Therefore, scientists need homogenous groups for consistent and reliable comparison. This is precisely what the concept MENTAL DISORDER affords.

Furthermore, an explication of MENTAL DISORDER may help us settle whether some controversial cases and types of mental disorders should count as such. To elaborate, claiming that something falls under a certain concept without having a definition for it is often unproblematic. For any given concept, there are uncontroversial, either real or hypothetical, cases in which our conceptual intuitions (or our pre-theoretical beliefs) pull distinctly in one direction and do not differ significantly from those of other people. In these cases, we do not need to refer to an explicit definition to justify our judgment, as our conceptual intuitions tend to suffice. However, there are also controversial cases in which our conceptual intuitions pull in different directions, or we have no intuitions to begin with. In these cases, our conceptual intuitions are not informative enough to settle disagreements. An explicit definition of the concept in question may help us settle controversial cases.

Ascriptions of mental disorder to individual cases are often contested, as intuitions about which cases fall under MENTAL DISORDER can differ widely. An explication of MENTAL DISORDER may help us settle the question of whether some putative cases of mental disorder should be treated as such. An explication may achieve this by providing the relevant *dimensions* by which these phenomena can be evaluated, case by case. For instance, some people may not share the intuition that Nives had a mental disorder, despite my assertion in the Introduction that she did. An explication of MENTAL DISORDER may put us in a better position to settle this dispute.

Many seemingly putative types of mental disorder are also contested. For instance, the categories of skin picking, gender dysphoria, premenstrual dysphoric disorder, binge-eating disorder, or disruptive mood dysregulation disorder are included in the fifth edition of the *Diagnostic and Statistical Manual of Mental Disorders (DSM-5)* (APA 2013), and yet these categories are at the center of much controversy (see Wakefield 2013, 2016). We may also question the inclusion of some categories, such as gambling addiction, given the exclusion of other, similar, categories, such as sex addiction. In addition, some have claimed that borderline, antisocial, histrionic, and narcissistic personality disorders are not mental disorders, but, instead, should be considered moral "disorders" or types of moral failures (see Boorse 2011 for an overview). According to this line of reasoning, the aforementioned personality disorders reflect a confusion between moral judgments and judgments about mental disorder. For similar reasons, some people hold that pedophilia, voyeurism, exhibitionism, or frotteurism should not be regarded as types of mental disorders (see Boorse 2011 for an overview). There is also a discussion over grief and mental disorder. Stephen Wilkinson (2000), for instance, argues that the exclusion of statistically normal grief is unjustified and arbitrary. He does not argue that we should consider grief to be a mental disorder, but only that, so far, we do not have sufficient reasons to think that we should not consider grief to fall under that concept.

What should we count as a mental disorder as opposed to, for example, a distressing deviation from social, moral, or other standards? An explication of MENTAL DISORDER may help us settle this question, for instance, by restricting the potential candidates, reducing potential inconsistencies and arbitrariness in a highly contested field.

1.2.2 *Practical or Normative Purposes*

There are also important practical, or normative, purposes for which we should use the concept MENTAL DISORDER.[6] Some of them actually explain our scientific interest in the phenomena in question. Furthermore, many significant and wide-ranging decisions depend on whether one considers an individual to have a mental disorder.

Most notably, having a mental disorder provides the affected individual with a *pro tanto* reason to seek psychiatric or psychotherapeutic treatment, and if such treatment is easily accessible to them, they may be justified to believe that they *should* seek it. Thus, MENTAL DISORDER may help us settle disputes over whether some individuals should seek psychiatric or psychotherapeutic treatment. It should be emphasized that having a mental disorder provides the affected individual with only a *pro tanto* reason to seek treatment of a certain type. It does not provide them with *sufficient* or *decisive* reason to do so because they may have other *pro tanto* reasons that count against, or outweigh, doing so. For example, an individual with a specific phobia of spiders might not have sufficient reason to seek psychiatric or psychotherapeutic treatment if the chances are low that they will be confronted with their fear and the costs of treatment are high. Thus, having a mental disorder, by itself, does not rationally oblige or require an individual to seek psychiatric or psychotherapeutic treatment.

Having a mental disorder also provides other people than the affected individual with a *pro tanto* reason to act in a certain way. On occasion, other people have a *pro tanto* reason to (partly) exempt or excuse an individual with a mental disorder from certain social, legal, or moral obligations, and may even have a reason to help them in some way. For instance, we should not (normatively) expect individuals with a mental disorder—such as major depressive disorder, say—to cope with the same workload or to provide the same emotional support to their loved ones, as individuals without a mental disorder (if we can expect them to work or provide emotional support at all).

Of course, not all disorders, mental or bodily, may justify exempting or excusing an individual from such obligations. For example, we do not extend the same types of exemptive considerations to individuals with minor bodily disorders, such as small injuries like paper cuts, or minor viral infections like a cough. Nevertheless, individuals with mental (or bodily) disorders often are, and should be, entitled to special consideration. In many societies, individuals with mental disorders are legally entitled to particular economic rights, such as social benefits, sick leave with compensation, publicly funded health care, or medical insurance reimbursement, and they are entitled as such in virtue of their having a mental disorder.

Furthermore, some individuals with a mental disorder are considered to have diminished responsibility when having committed a crime or may be considered to lack criminal responsibility altogether because of their having a (severe) mental disorder. Consider, for instance, the German Criminal Code ("StGB"). Section 20, "Lack of criminal responsibility due to mental disorder" of the StGB regulates cases in which an individual lacks criminal responsibility:

> Whoever, at the time of the commission of the offence, is incapable of appreciating the unlawfulness of their actions or of acting in accordance with any such appreciation due to a pathological mental disorder, a profound disturbance of consciousness or intellectual disability or any other serious mental disorder is deemed to act without guilt.
>
> (Federal Ministry of Justice and Consumer Protection, n.d.)

Section 21 of the StGB regulates "diminished responsibility":

> If the offender's capacity to appreciate the unlawfulness of the act or to act in accordance with any such appreciation is substantially diminished at the time of the commission of the offence due to one of the reasons indicated in section 20, the penalty may be mitigated pursuant to section 49 (1).
>
> (Federal Ministry of Justice and Consumer Protection, n.d.)

It is worth emphasizing that, in order to be (partly) exempt from criminal responsibility, it is necessary that the individual in question (a) lacks the ability to understand the difference between what is legally right and wrong, or (b) lacks the ability to act in accordance with the understanding of the difference between what is legally right and wrong.

In sum, we need the concept of MENTAL DISORDER to help us settle disputes over (1) whether an individual should seek psychiatric or psychotherapeutic treatment, and (2) whether they should be (partly) exempt or excused from certain social, legal, or moral obligations. If an individual has a mental disorder, they will have a pro tanto reason to seek psychiatric or psychotherapeutic treatment. Likewise, other people will have a *pro tanto* reason to (partly) exempt or excuse the affected individual from certain social, legal, or moral obligations, or to help them in some way.

However, some authors argue that the concept MENTAL DISORDER does not help us settle the aforementioned normative questions. Hesslow (1993), for example, argues that the relationships between disorder (or, in his terminology, "disease") and medical treatment, medical insurance, special rights, and moral or legal responsibility, are not straightforward. On his view, having a disorder does not, by itself, necessitate any of these normative consequences and other important conditions are connected to them as well. Having a disorder does not give the affected individual decisive reason to seek medical treatment, and an individual may also have other *pro tanto* reasons to consult a physician than having a disorder (for example, regarding pregnancy, contraception, or similar). In light of this, Hesslow (1993) argues that a DISORDER concept cannot help us settle the question of who should seek medical treatment. Furthermore, according to Hesslow, the DISORDER concept is itself a "straightjacket" (1993, 1) from which we should free ourselves. The same argument applies *mutatis mutandis* to the case of MENTAL DISORDER.

However, I would contend that Hesslow's conclusions are unnecessarily strong. First, MENTAL DISORDER does help us settle the aforementioned normative questions, even if it might not do so decisively. It is clear that when asking *who* has a *pro tanto* reason to seek psychiatric or psychotherapeutic treatment, our answer should be those individuals with mental disorders. Hesslow's argument that having a mental disorder does not give an individual decisive reason and that there may be other individuals who also have *pro tanto* reasons to seek psychiatric or psychotherapeutic treatment, while correct, does not render this answer unhelpful or uninformative. Hesslow's analysis merely shows that the question of whether an individual should seek psychiatric or psychotherapeutic treatment does not depend on the condition of having a mental disorder *alone*.

I argue further, contrary to Hesslow, that the concept MENTAL DISORDER is very informative. The presence of mental disorder does not imply a range of vague normative consequences, but highly specific ones. Having a mental disorder gives the individual a *pro tanto* reason to seek *psychiatric or psychotherapeutic* treatment, not just any type of response. To take an analogous case, we may ask who is entitled to praise. A reasonable response would be to say it is those individuals who exemplify bravery. However, individuals who are just, for example, also deserve praise. One may conclude from this that it is therefore irrelevant to know whether someone is brave or just because in both cases the individuals deserve praise. However, I argue that it is still relevant to ask who deserves praise, as the answer may differ depending on what, exactly, we want to know. If we only want to know whether some individual deserves praise, it is sufficient to know that they have done something good. However, if we want to know what type of praise they deserve, knowing that they have done something good will not suffice. In this case, we need to know more, such as whether they were specifically brave or just, or in what respect they have done something good.

As with the case of praise, it is true that types of mental conditions other than mental disorders call for responses as well, but they are not completely unrelated to mental disorders. Many types of mental conditions may be a result of, or consequently lead to, a mental disorder itself. For example, it is controversial whether early psychotherapeutic or pharmacological interventions for individuals exposed to trauma are effective in preventing them from incurring trauma- or stressor-related disorders. Some guidelines state that early preventive interventions may be helpful, while a more recent review of the empirical data suggests that the recommendations offered in these guidelines are insufficiently supported by the evidence (see Ursano et al. 2004, Forbes et al. 2010). The question arises as to why early psychotherapeutic or pharmacological interventions are offered to individuals who do not have a mental disorder in the first place. The rationale behind the recommendations seems to be that being exposed to trauma puts an individual at risk of incurring a mental disorder such as a trauma- or stressor-related disorder. If it turns out that they are not at risk, we would not believe that a psychotherapeutic or pharmacological intervention is needed.

1.2.3 Actual Usage

The actual technical usage of MENTAL DISORDER is captured in the two most influential classification systems for mental disorders: the *DSM-5* and the *ICD-11*. The *DSM-5*, mentioned earlier, was issued by the American Psychiatric Association (APA) in 2013. The *ICD-11* is the 11th, and most recent, revision of the *International Classification of Diseases for Mortality and Morbidity Statistics*, which was issued by the World Health Organization (WHO) in 2019. Whereas the *DSM-5* lists 19 broadly defined categories of mental disorder (with the further residual category of "other mental disorders"), the *ICD-11* lists 18 broad categories that cover mental, behavioral, or neurodevelopmental disorders, as well as five closely related ones.

The categories in the *DSM-5* and the *ICD-11* have significant overlap. While some of the categories have slightly different names, these groupings aim to grasp, more or less, the same type of phenomena. For instance, the category "trauma- and stressor-related disorders" attempts to capture the same experiences as the category "disorders specifically associated with stress." We may additionally see similarities between the categories of "somatic symptom and related disorders" and "disorders of bodily distress or bodily experience." Further overlap may be noted in cases where, using one system of categorization, a particular classification separates two types of phenomena which, in the other system, are included under one, more general category. Here are some examples:

a The *ICD-11* category "catatonia" is subsumed more or less under the *DSM-5* category "schizophrenia spectrum and other psychotic disorders."
b The *ICD-11* categories "impulse control disorders" and "disruptive behavior or dissocial disorders" are subsumed more or less under the *DSM-5* category "disruptive, impulse-control, and conduct disorders."
c The *ICD-11* category "factitious disorder" is subsumed under the *DSM-5* category "somatic symptom and related disorders."
d The *DSM-5* categories "bipolar and related disorders" and "depressive disorders" are subsumed more or less under the *ICD-11* category "mood disorders."

The most significant difference between the two systems is that the *ICD-11* does not categorize "sleep-wake disorders," "sexual dysfunctions," and "gender incongruence" primarily as "mental, behavioral, or neurodevelopmental disorders," but, rather, as disorders of other types. Owing to these differences, I argue that the status of these three types of phenomena is more controversial than that of other presumed mental disorders.

1.3 Adequacy Conditions

To systematically evaluate an existing conception of MENTAL DISORDER, we must first specify a set of conditions that any comprehensive explication of MENTAL DISORDER, for the aforementioned purposes, will have to meet in order for it to adequately capture its subject matter.[7] I propose the following four adequacy conditions.[8] Any explication of MENTAL DISORDER will have to

1 clarify the distinction between MENTAL DISORDER and MENTAL HEALTH;
2 clarify the distinction between MENTAL DISORDER and BODILY DISORDER (or, at a minimum, clarify the concept of the MENTAL in MENTAL DISORDER);
3 clarify the relation between having a mental disorder and violating some non-medical—say, social, legal, or moral—norm; and

4 make intelligible what it is about having a mental disorder that justifies certain normative consequences such as

  a giving the affected individual a *pro tanto* reason to seek psychiatric or psychotherapeutic treatment (if available); and
  b giving others a *pro tanto* reason to (partly) exempt or excuse the affected individual from certain social, legal, or moral obligations, or to help them in some way (if possible).

In the following, I will elaborate on each of these adequacy conditions in turn.

1.3.1 Mental Disorder versus Mental Health

The first adequacy condition concerns the conceptual distinction between MENTAL DISORDER and MENTAL HEALTH. Any explication of MENTAL DISORDER will have to

  a include clear cases of pathological mental conditions, exclude clear cases of non-pathological mental conditions, avoid absurd consequences; and
  b include as many of the overlapping categories of mental disorder listed in the *DSM-5* and *ICD-11* as possible.

With regard to (a), any explication must rely on particular cases that (i) clearly do (or should) and (ii) clearly do not (or should not) fall under the concept-to-be-explicated. Otherwise, the resulting definition would be a purely stipulated one. Any explication will therefore have to capture the aforementioned cases accordingly.

With regard to (b), despite the requirement of any conservative explication of MENTAL DISORDER to be as consistent with our current diagnostic systems as possible, any explication should also allow for revision. The fact that the method of explication allows for revision is useful because it allows our definition to be refined as our scientific understanding of controversial categories of mental disorder in our current diagnostic systems develops. Nevertheless, we, as theorists, should not make major revisions without good independent reasons.

In addition, let me mention a further adequacy condition; one which I shall *not* discuss in this book but which is nevertheless important to keep in mind. Any comprehensive view of MENTAL DISORDER should also be able to take a stance on the problems that arise from *vagueness*. The term "mental disorder" seems to be vague (see Keil, Keuck, and Hauswald 2017). "Vague" is a technical term, with vagueness being a semantic property of linguistic expressions (Keil, Keuck, and Hauswald 2017, 6). To claim that "mental disorder" is semantically vague is to claim that it does not draw a sharp boundary between its extension and anti-extension. This lack of distinct boundary gives rise to so-called borderline cases. A case may be called borderline when it is semantically unclear whether it falls under the concept MENTAL DISORDER or not. However, semantic vagueness should not be confused with epistemic uncertainty (Keil, Keuck, and Hauswald 2017, 7). We may not *know*, for a particular case, whether it falls under a certain concept because we simply do not have all the relevant facts to make such a judgment. For instance, one might be uncertain whether an individual has an addictive disorder related to alcohol because one does not know how much alcohol they drink. This case is epistemically uncertain, but it is not necessarily a borderline case in the semantic sense.

Now we need ascriptions of mental disorder to apply categorically, and yet "mental disorder" appears to be semantically vague. This raises two problems:

1 *The Problem of Drawing the Line*: Where should we draw the line between pathological and non-pathological mental conditions? Where is the threshold?[9]
2 *The Problem of Borderline Cases*: Wherever the line is drawn, it is likely to yield borderline cases. How, then, should we deal with them?

Returning to our example of addictive disorder related to alcohol, we may ask at which point on the continuum of "drinking alcohol" do cases of non-pathological drinking stop and cases of disorder arise. Suppose that we draw the line at "drinking alcohol every day." Why should we draw the line there and not at, for example, "drinking alcohol six days a week"? But if we were to move our line to include as a disorder "drinking alcohol six days a week," it would be unclear where to place a person who drinks, for example, only five to six days a week. Any comprehensive view of MENTAL DISORDER should be able to take a stance on these problems. Since this is a large topic, I will leave it for another time.

1.3.2 Mental Disorder versus Bodily Disorder

In both ordinary language and in science, we distinguish between bodily (or somatic) disorders, such as diabetes, cancer, and viral infections, and mental disorders, such as panic disorder, obsessive-compulsive disorder, and major depressive disorder. One might ask: what, if anything, do these types of disorders have in common and what is the difference between them? In other words, we may ask how exactly the concepts BODILY DISORDER and MENTAL DISORDER relate to each other. For instance, we may consider (a) both to be subcategories of the more general category DISORDER, or (b) MENTAL DISORDER to be a subcategory of BODILY DISORDER, or (c) both to be distinct categories. Any *analysis* of MENTAL DISORDER must capture this distinction by specifying the conditions in light of which it is made.

An *explication* of MENTAL DISORDER, however, does not necessarily have to capture this distinction, unless the distinction itself is useful for the priorly defined purposes. Given that the project of this book is to provide an explication, not an analysis, I must first elaborate on whether the distinction between BODILY DISORDER and MENTAL DISORDER is of any use to the aforementioned scientific or normative purposes. If it is, then the explication of MENTAL DISORDER will have to clarify at a minimum the concept of the MENTAL in MENTAL DISORDER. (Developing a positive explication of the concept BODILY DISORDER is not required.) If the distinction is of no use, then an explication of MENTAL DISORDER may nevertheless help us explain why we often make such a distinction, despite its lack of contribution to the aforementioned purposes.

I argue that we should explore the distinction between BODILY DISORDER and MENTAL DISORDER because the distinction may have *practical* consequences. For instance, there are certain types of therapies, for example, cognitive-behavioral therapy, psychoanalysis, or conversational therapy, which are suitable for treating some mental disorders, but do not appear appropriate for treating (merely) bodily ones. This suggests that our choices of treatment will differ depending on whether a disorder is deemed to be, primarily, a mental one or a (merely) bodily one. Perhaps, the best way to treat, for example, a somatic symptom disorder is different than the best way to treat a (merely) bodily disorder with similar symptoms.

There are also *theoretical* reasons to explore the distinction between BODILY DISORDER and MENTAL DISORDER. It is not clear that the distinction between "pathological" and "non-pathological" mental conditions can be equated with the distinction between "pathological" and "non-pathological" bodily conditions. One might argue that the concepts MENTAL DISORDER and BODILY DISORDER should not be understood as two subcategories of a more general category DISORDER. Instead, one might argue that the meaning of the term "pathological" should be understood *relative* to the structures of (a) the body and (b) the mind. If the structures of the body and the mind are, in fact, different, then one might argue that the term "pathological" has two different meanings. Therefore, exploring the distinction between BODILY DISORDER and MENTAL DISORDER could also help us explicate the relation between MENTAL DISORDER and MENTAL HEALTH.

1.3.3 *Mental Disorder versus Deviances from Social, Legal, or Moral Norms*

There is a difference between individuals having a mental disorder and individuals merely violating a social, legal, or moral norm. This is because for an individual to have a mental disorder, it is generally not necessary that they violate any of these types of norms (except in some mental disorders such as "conduct disorder"). For example, an individual might be both depressed and highly compliant to moral and legal norms. They may also reliably meet the expectations that come with their various social roles. Furthermore, violating social, legal, or moral norms is not sufficient for having a mental disorder; an individual might be an unfriendly and deceptive scam artist but these features alone do not justify appropriately labeling this individual as having a mental disorder.

Nevertheless, having a mental disorder and violating social, legal, or moral norms are not completely unrelated phenomena. Szasz suggests that "[i]n actual contemporary social usage, the finding of a mental illness is made by establishing a deviance in behavior from certain psychosocial, ethical, or legal norms" (1960, 115). This claim can be interpreted in two ways: (a) certain types of mental disorder are *defined* by a deviance from a social, legal, or moral norm, or (b) social, legal, or moral norms may play an *epistemological* role in finding out about whether a certain individual has a mental disorder of some type. By examining the *DSM-5* we find both interpretations present in our actual technical usage of MENTAL DISORDER.

Some diagnostic criteria appear to either explicitly or implicitly refer to some of these norms. For instance, in the *DSM-5*, one criterion for "conduct disorder" is a

> repetitive and persistent pattern of behavior in which the basic rights of other or major age-appropriate societal norms or rules are violated, as manifested by the presence of at least three of the following 15 criteria in the past 12 months from any categories below, with at least one criterion present in the past 6 months.
>
> (2013, 469)

A diagnosis of conduct disorder may be evidenced by particular "patterns" of norm violation, such as, for example, when an individual "[o]ften bullies, threatens, or intimidates others," "[h]as stolen items of nontrivial value without confronting a victim (e.g. shoplifting, but without breaking and entering; forgery)," and/or "[o]ften lies to obtain goods or favors to avoid obligations (i.e., 'cons' others)." In cases like these, the norms in question play a defining role, and it is also through witnessing the violations of such norms that we gain knowledge about whether an individual has a conduct disorder.

When it comes to cases of mental disorder and norm violation, Gary Watson (2004) has pointed out an interesting paradox in our intuitions around extreme evil and moral responsibility. He argues that, while we tend to condemn individuals who commit extremely evil acts for their actions, we do not tend to hold them to be our moral interlocutors. In the most extreme cases of moral evildoing, Watson claims, we frequently make the assumption that "something must have gone wrong in the developmental histories of these individuals, if not in their socialization, then 'in them'—in their genes or brains" (2004, 247). Thus, according to our moral intuitions, an extreme violation of a moral norm indicates that the individual necessarily has a mental disorder. If true, this could have interesting consequences for ascriptions of criminal responsibility. If an individual who commits extremely evil actions necessarily has a mental disorder, because their actions are so reprehensible that there must be some explanation for these actions (that being having a mental disorder) beyond that individual's control, then such an individual might not be fully criminally responsible for their actions. However, one must be careful when raising such claims because, in fact, having a mental disorder is rarely sufficient for a diminishment of criminal responsibility.

Based on these considerations, any explication of MENTAL DISORDER should capture the fact that (1) in general, violating a social, legal, or moral norm is neither necessary nor sufficient for having a mental disorder (and *vice versa*), and yet (2) for some types of mental disorders, the violation of a social, legal, or moral norm plays a defining role. Furthermore, (3) social, legal, or moral norms may play an epistemological role in the diagnosis of some types of mental disorders. In addition, (4) an explication should also offer some help in deciding whether we are justified in believing that the worst moral evildoers must have a mental disorder.

1.3.4 Normative Purposes

In Section 1.2, I claimed that we do not categorize mental conditions as pathological or non-pathological purely for the purpose of categorization. And I highlighted that having a mental disorder has the following normative consequences:

a having a mental disorder provides the affected individual with a *pro tanto* reason to seek psychiatric or psychotherapeutic treatment (if available), and
b having a mental disorder provides others with a *pro tanto* reason to (partly) exempt or excuse an individual with a mental disorder from certain social, legal, or moral obligations, or to help them in some way (if possible).

In certain social, legal, and moral contexts, it is justified, and may even be required, to treat individuals with mental disorders differently, in some respect, to individuals without a mental disorder. When this is the case, it is the fact that the individual in question has a mental disorder that justifies the difference in treatment. This is not to say that (a) different treatment is always justified, or that (b) we are morally permitted, on any occasion, to treat individuals with mental disorders inhumanely, or in any way that is degrading or without respect. Historically, people have marginalized, neglected, abused, and inflicted violence upon those with mental disorders, using the power and authority psychiatry can afford. In the present day, the civil rights of individuals with mental disorder are still not always respected as they should be. Such abuses are not, and never were, morally permitted.

Instead, I argue that "different treatment" in the case of mental disorder entails treatment with *greater care*. For instance, an individual with a depressive disorder deserves—in the moral sense of the term—to receive psychiatric or psychotherapeutic treatment and be treated by other people with greater sensitivity.[10] It seems morally just that these individuals be entitled to certain economic and legal rights, and be excused from certain social obligations. Nevertheless, Stephen Morse points out that "[t]reating people with mental disorder specially is a two-edged sword. Failing to do so when appropriate is unjust, but the opposite is demeaning, stigmatizing, and paternalistic" (2011, 886). In light of this, it is necessary to develop a set of criteria that determine under what conditions different treatments may be justified. Specifying these criteria, however, would constitute a wholly different project that I cannot concern myself with here. Nevertheless, any explication of MENTAL DISORDER for normative purposes will have to account for the fact that having a mental disorder *generally* has some social, legal, and moral consequences, as well as make intelligible why this is the case.

1.4 Why Explication?

In the Introduction, I claimed that we need a definition of MENTAL DISORDER for certain scientific and normative purposes.[11] One might question why explication should be the method of choice for developing such a definition. In this section, I will argue that we should pursue an explication because only explication is concerned explicitly with purposes, and only purposes can help us settle disagreements as to whether certain mental conditions should fall under MENTAL DISORDER in a non-arbitrary way (to the extent that this is possible).

I will elaborate on this argument by first discussing a couple of objections. Critic A might object that explication gets things back-to-front; we should not answer the question of what mental disorders *are* by first defining MENTAL DISORDER so that it fits our purposes. Rather, we should proceed the other way around by first identifying what mental disorders are and then evaluating if, and under which circumstances, having a mental disorder fits certain purposes. To put this simply, we should first identify the structure of the world and then consider the structure in relation to our purposes and normative consequences. We should not *make* categories but aim to identify and represent the categories that already exist in the world.

Furthermore, critic A might argue that engaging in a conceptual analysis of MENTAL DISORDER would also be misguided because this method cannot help us identify what mental disorders really are, but only what people believe mental disorders to be (see Murphy 2006). In light of these objections, critic A might argue that a more appropriate project would be an empirical investigation of the phenomena in question. Because according to critic A, only empirical investigation aims at identifying the structure of the world as it really is, independent of its investigators, or, in other words, aims at "carving nature at its joints."[12]

I will respond to critic A's argument by discussing the methods of (1) empirical investigation and (2) conceptual analysis, in turn.

1.4.1 Empirical Investigation

Dominic Murphy provides an initial outline of how we might develop a definition of MENTAL DISORDER by means of an empirical investigation:

> Our investigation of mental illness should respect certain core examples: if schizophrenia and major depression are not mental illnesses, then it is hard to know what a mental illness could be. So, I imagine psychiatry proceeding via ostension, in the sense that we start with core examples, try to explain them and explain things like them, then extend the explanatory structure that the ostensive approach generates as far as it should go.
>
> (2006, 62)

Drawing on Murphy, we may say that developing a definition of MENTAL DISORDER by means of an empirical investigation will involve the following three steps: (1) determining a set of core types of phenomena, (2) describing and/or explaining these core types of phenomena, and (3) extending the descriptions and/or explanations to other similar types of phenomena "as far as they should go."

This characterization reveals that even a definition of MENTAL DISORDER based on an empirical investigation importantly depends on a prior categorization of certain types of phenomena *as* mental disorders. In order to get an empirical investigation of the ground, we need to know what to investigate or, at least, where to look. In order to proceed, then, we will need to provide, at least, an ostensive (or extensional) definition of MENTAL DISORDER by pointing out some phenomena, of which we can say definitively, "These [phenomena] are mental disorders." Therefore, any definition of MENTAL DISORDER developed by empirical investigation must start with at least some (pre-)theoretical beliefs about which phenomena clearly fall, or should fall, under that concept. Given this, even an empirical definition must depend on a set of core types of phenomena we believe to be mental disorders. This is why I argue the project of empirical investigation cannot be pursued independently of the use of some concepts.

Moreover, in order to develop a general definition of MENTAL DISORDER, merely pointing out a few core types of phenomena—say, schizophrenia and depression—will not be sufficient. Our initial set of clear cases will have to be extended to include other types of phenomena as well. However, it is not evident which new phenomena our set should include. According to Murphy (2006), we should extend our set of cases to types of phenomena that are similar. But this answer is ultimately dissatisfying because similarity is always similarity *in some respect*. Individuals can be similar to one another with respect to a range of different properties, such as their psychological, biological, physical, chemical, or other types of properties. Furthermore, any two entities may be said to be similar to each other in some respect, even if their only shared property is that they are both entities. Murphy's criteria for generalization raises the question, therefore, as to which characteristics are relevant for determining which other types of phenomena should be added to the initial set of mental disorders. This question cannot be answered by purely empirical means, as it is not possible to observe which types of phenomena should be added, nor is it clear which observations we would need to make in order to determine that. This question needs to be settled in light of our reasons, and the reasons we have may differ depending on the purposes for which we (should) use the concept MENTAL DISORDER.

To put it differently, we investigate the world through empirical means and aim to generate useful categories and classifications. In principle, multiple sets of categories and classifications may be generated. Given that there are multiple options for creating categories and classifications, the normative question of which categories and classification(s) we should create applies. The answer will depend, in part, on the purposes for which we (should) use them. There may be more or less comprehensive, coherent, clear, simple, arbitrary, and useful classifications. Given certain empirical findings, certain classifications may turn out to be empirically better or worse along some of these dimensions. Nevertheless, the dimensions themselves by which we assess our classifications cannot be determined by empirical means alone; if, and to what degree, a system of classification is comprehensive, coherent, clear, simple, and non-arbitrary will depend, in part, on the purposes for which we (should) use them, as well as the purposes on which their quality is judged.[13]

Critic A may try to defend their position by arguing that our categories and classifications should enable us to articulate truths, pointing out that the main aim of scientific classifications is to capture something true. However, as Sally Haslanger notes, "an unconstrained search for truth would yield chaos, not theory; truths are too easy to come by, there are too many of them" (2000, 35). Simply put, truth is not enough. To get at the heart of this point, consider why we make classifications of mental and bodily disorders specifically, and not of, for instance, the various shapes of the "pinkie toe" (that is, the little toe). After all, a classification of the shapes of pinkie toes would also enable us to articulate truths, namely, truths about the various shapes of pinkie toes. The reason we don't make such classifications, but do so for the case of disorders, is because we believe that having a mental or bodily disorder makes (or should make) a difference in some scientific and normative contexts, whereas an individual's shape of pinkie toe does not, or should not. It is therefore important to theorize about the purposes for which we use our concepts in order to constrain empirical investigation because an endless pursuit of truth would result in too many (equivalent) classifications of phenomena.

1.4.2 Conceptual Analysis

If a definition of a concept, F, can be obtained by analyzing our actual correct ascriptions of the property *F*, it may appear reasonable to first define our concept through conceptual analysis before evaluating the normative consequences our actual concept MENTAL DISORDER has in respect to our various purposes for using this concept.[14]

Before discussing this proposal, let me first clarify a misunderstanding about conceptual analysis. Conceptual analysis presupposes that there are correct and incorrect ascriptions of mental disorder. But one might argue that this relies on a false assumption, given that the set of phenomena we call "mental disorder" has changed markedly over time. For example, the list of diagnoses used by psychiatrists has both expanded and contracted over the decades, with new categories being included while others are expelled. Drapetomania, the "urge to flee from slavery," was believed to be a category of mental disorder in the 19th century.[15] Hysteria used to be a diagnosis for women in distress.[16] Homosexuality was removed as a category of mental disorder with the *DSM-III R* (1987). Asperger's syndrome was removed with the *DSM-5* (APA 2013), or, rather, it was integrated into the single broad category called "autism spectrum disorder." New disorder categories such as skin picking, gender dysphoria, premenstrual dysphoric disorder, binge-eating disorder, and disruptive mood dysregulation disorder (children showing persistent bad temper with bursts of rage) have been a part of our classificatory system since 2013. In light of these changes, a critic might ask: don't these changes indicate that there are *no* correct ascriptions of mental disorder after all?

I would contend that they do not. It is true that there have been significant changes in what we call "mental disorder." But this does not imply
that there are no correct ascriptions of mental disorder. It is compatible to
claim both that the set of phenomena we call "mental disorder" has
changed and that there are, nevertheless, correct (and incorrect) ascriptions of mental disorder. The proponent of conceptual analysis has at least
two options to explain how this might be the case.

First, one might say that the concept associated with the term "mental
disorder" changed with each decision about which phenomena should be
called "mental disorder." On this view, individuals who lived before 1986
simply meant something different by "mental disorder" from what we
mean today when they said, for instance, "homosexuality is a mental
disorder." A plausible account of this difference might be that, at this
time, "mental disorder" used to be defined, roughly, as "a condition that
people in a society condemn," unlike today where it is defined as, roughly,
"a condition that is in a psychiatric or psychological sense 'not okay' or
'not in order.'"

Second, one might argue that people in the past were simply mistaken
about which phenomena fell under the concept associated with the term
"mental disorder," which, itself, has not changed throughout history. It is
possible, for example, that by "mental disorder" we have always meant
something like "a condition that is in a psychiatric or psychological sense
'not okay' or 'not in order.'" On this view, people who believed in the past,
or still believe today, that homosexuality falls under the concept MENTAL
DISORDER have always falsely believed that. This may be possible if they
were mistaken about what exactly it means to be "in a psychiatric or psychological sense 'not okay' or 'not in order.'"

In sum, it is either the case that people in the past said something true by
the statement "homosexuality is a mental disorder," but stated something
other than what we mean by the same statement today, or they stated the
same as we do today, but the statement was flatly false in the past and
continues to be false today. In either case, that the phenomena we call
"mental disorder" has changed does not imply that there are no correct
ascriptions of mental disorder. What the previous example shows is that
the correctness of our ascription covaries with the concept that is associated with the term "mental disorder." Different concepts associated with
the term "mental disorder" yield different correct ascriptions of mental
disorder and *vice versa*. The project of conceptual analysis may become
more complex in light of this, but it may be broadly understood as the
project of revealing the concept(s) associated with the term "mental disorder" by analyzing how we use the term "mental disorder" (and other similar terms) in colloquial and/or technical contexts today and/or how we
used them in the past.

Now, in principle, there is nothing wrong with engaging in a conceptual analysis of MENTAL DISORDER first and then evaluating which normative consequences are attached to it second. However, there is something that conceptual analysis cannot give us: clarification. Given that the field to which MENTAL DISORDER applies is contested, it would be fruitful for a definition of MENTAL DISORDER to give us the means to settle these disagreements. The method of conceptual analysis cannot give us that because the definition it provides needs to reflect our actual usage, and if our actual use of a concept includes cases in which it is unclear whether the phenomenon falls under that concept, an analysis of that concept must also reflect that unclarity. By contrast, an explication of MENTAL DISORDER would allow us to change our concepts to make them amenable to our purposes. Given its potential to resolve conflict, an explication of MENTAL DISORDER may be more fruitful than a conceptual analysis.

In addition, the method of conceptual analysis does not address whether we should continue to use our current MENTAL DISORDER concept. In principle, we can change our concepts, for example, by changing the purposes for which we make ascriptions of these concepts in the first place. This is to say that we should not take the set of phenomena that we currently consider falling under MENTAL DISORDER for granted. Our current MENTAL DISORDER concept has no priority over other possible MENTAL DISORDER concepts simply in virtue of being the one we actually and presently use. So, it is an open question whether we should continue to use our current MENTAL DISORDER concept or not. I would argue that, in the end, we care about the purposes for which we use certain concepts. If this is the real issue, then, arguably, we should address it directly instead of making a detour via conceptual analysis.

To summarize, we use concepts, and in doing so, we create categories and classifications of the world, rather than discovering them. We do not make them simply for the sake of classification, but we do so with the intention of these concepts serving certain purposes. It is these purposes in virtue of which we can evaluate different categories and classifications. We can assess whether a certain category or classification is fruitful with regard to the purposes for which it was made and whether it was made for good purposes in the first place.

Conceptual analysis, empirical investigation, and explication are different projects with different merits. The method we should choose depends on the goals we are interested in. Given that we need a concept that serves certain scientific and normative purposes and helps us settle certain disagreements, explication appears to be the best method for this project.

Before continuing, let me address a concern from Eric Matthews, who raises the following objection to the project of explicating MENTAL DISORDER:

> [The method] is also somewhat circular. For, to be able to set out the goals that we have in classifying some people as mentally disordered, we *already* have to know which persons we so classify, and so what is meant by calling them "mentally disordered."
>
> (2009, 56)

It is true that in order to explicate a concept, F, we must assume that at least some phenomena fall under F, meaning we must have some pre-theoretical beliefs about what we mean by calling them "F." However, we have to start somewhere, regardless of which method exactly we pursue. Otherwise, we could simply stipulate a definition of "F." I, therefore, agree that explication involves some circularity, but circularity need not be problematic or uninformative. Explication does not require that we start with a complete extension of F or a full understanding of the meaning of "F." Therefore, if we have a minimal consensus on which phenomena should fall under F, as well as some minimal shared understanding of the meaning of "F," we may still proceed with an explication.

Notes

1 Strawson (1992, 7) gives the following analogy:

> Just as the grammarian, and especially the model modern grammarian, labours to produce a systematic account of the structure of rules which we effortlessly observe in speaking grammatically, so the philosopher labours to produce a systematic account of the general conceptual structure of which our daily practice shows us to have a tacit and unconscious mastery.

2 Not all methods fit neatly into this distinction. The "Canberra plan," for instance, is a project in which we (1) assemble folk platitudes about a certain subject matter, (2) discover what in the world occupies that role, and (3) identify the subject matter with what in the world occupies the role (Lewis 1994, Jackson 1998). The Canberra plan could be understood as a project that begins as an analysis and then proceeds as an explication, and that presumably, aims to "carve nature at its joints," or, in other words, aims to identify the concept-independent structure of reality.

3 Typically, we do not have to analyze technical concepts, as they tend to be stipulated by the scientific user or community of scientific users.

4 In *pure stipulation*, by contrast, we introduce a new concept from scratch.

5 Brülde denies that we need a definition for theoretical purposes because mental disorder is not a natural kind, and "it is unlikely that any of the medical sciences need a category of mental disorder" (2010, 20). I argue that the sciences related to mental disorder *are* in need of a category of mental disorder, but that this does not presuppose that mental disorder is a natural kind.

6 See Brülde (2010, 21) for a discussion on different candidates for appropriate normative purposes, such as a method to "help us decide who is entitled to publicly funded health care or medical insurance reimbursement" or "help us determine who is entitled to sick leave with compensation." I broadly agree with Brülde's view that "the primary practical purpose of a definition [of MENTAL

DISORDER] is that it should help us make better decisions" (2010, 21). However, I put forward a slightly different view in terms of which decisions are at stake.

7 I shall use "any explication of MENTAL DISORDER" as a shorthand for "any comprehensive explication of MENTAL DISORDER for the aforementioned purposes."

8 Brülde (2010, 27 ff.) lists the following adequacy conditions for a definition of MENTAL DISORDER: it should (1) be consistent with ordinary language; (2) explain why we regard most or all disorders as harmful; (3) be ideally general and coherent; (4) draw sharp boundaries between health and disorder; (5) be "practically applicable; it should be relatively easy in *practice* (not just in principle) to determine whether a certain condition is a mental disorder (as defined)"; (6) be as simple as possible; (7) be normatively adequate.

   I agree with (3), (6), and (7), but I do not mention (3) and (6) explicitly above because they apply to all explications. Because I am interested in a technical concept, I am not committed to conditions (1) and (2). Furthermore, I would argue that condition (4) is too much to ask of a philosophical explication. Moreover, explicating a concept, F, and giving epistemic criteria for determining what falls under F are two different projects. Because I am interested in the former project, I am not committed to condition (5) either.

9 I named this problem in reference to Schwartz (2007) who points out the same issue for biological function views of disorder.

10 For a normative justification of this point, see Daniels (2000, 2008, 2009) who argues that one key role of medical care is to protect one's right to equality of opportunity.

11 Someone might rightly ask why we should not pursue two explications, one of MENTAL DISORDER$_1$ for scientific and one of MENTAL DISORDER$_2$ for normative purposes. One problem with this suggestion is that it would lead to "coordination problems" (Cooper 2020, 151). Furthermore, the normative purposes are not independent from the scientific ones and, thus, we would be mistaken to believe that we should pursue two wholly independent projects.

12 It seems to be agreed upon that Plato (1952) stated it first in *Phaedrus* 265d–266a.

13 Furthermore, it is possible that what counts as "comprehensive," "coherent," "clear," "simple," and "non-arbitrary" is relative to our purposes as well.

14 See Nordby (2006), Lemoine (2013), and Schwartz (2014) for critiques of conceptual analysis in the medical realm.

15 The term "drapetomania" was coined by the physician Samuel A. Cartwright (1851). For a critical discussion, see Szasz (1971).

16 See Tasca et al. (2012) for a short history of hysteria and Szasz (1961) for a critical discussion.

References

American Psychiatric Association (APA). 1987. *Diagnostic and Statistical Manual of Mental Disorders: DSM-III-R*. Washington: American Psychiatric Association.

———. 2013. *Diagnostic and Statistical Manual of Mental Disorders: DSM-5*. Arlington: American Psychiatric Association.

Boorse, Christopher. 2011. "Concepts of Health and Disease." In *Philosophy of Medicine*, edited by Fred Gifford, 13–64. Munich: Elsevier.

Brülde, Bengt. 2010. "On Defining 'Mental Disorder': Purposes and Conditions of Adequacy." *Theoretical Medicine and Bioethics* 31 (1): 19–33.

Carnap, Rudolf. 1950. *Logical Foundations of Probability*. Chicago: University of Chicago Press.

Cartwright, Samuel A. 1851. "The Diseases and Physical Peculiarities of the Negro Race." *Southern Medical Reports* 2: 421–429.

Cooper, Rachel. 2020. "The Concept of Disorder Revisited: Robustly Value-Laden despite Change." *Aristotelian Society Supplementary* 94 (1): 141–161.

Daniels, Norman. 2000. "Normal Functioning and the Treatment-Enhancement Distinction." *Cambridge Quarterly of Healthcare Ethics* 9: 309–322.

———. 2008. *Just Health: Meeting Health Needs Fairly*. Cambridge: Cambridge University Press.

———. 2009. "Just Health: Replies and Further Thoughts." *Journal of Medical Ethics* 35: 36–41.

Federal Ministry of Justice and Consumer Protection. n.d. "German Criminal Code." Accessed April 3, 2023. http://www.gesetze-im-internet.de/index.html.

Forbes, David, Mark Creamer, Jonathan I. Bisson, Judith A Cohen, Bruce E. Crow, Edna B. Foa, Mathew J. Friedman, Terence M. Keane, Harold S. Kudler, and Robert J. Ursano. 2010. "A Guide to Guidelines for the Treatment of PTSD and Related Conditions." *Journal of Traumatic Stress* 23 (5): 537–552.

Haslanger, Sally. 2000. "Gender and Race: (What) Are They? (What) Do We Want Them to Be?" *Noûs* 34 (1): 31–55.

Hesslow, Germund. 1993. "Do We Need a Concept of Disease?" *Theoretical Medicine and Bioethics* 14 (1): 1–14.

Jackson, Frank. 1998. *From Metaphysics to Ethics: A Defense of Conceptual Analysis*. Oxford: Oxford University Press.

Keil, Geert, Lara Keuck, and Rico Hauswald, eds. 2017. *Vagueness in Psychiatry*. Oxford: Oxford University Press.

Lemoine, Maël. 2013. "Defining Disease beyond Conceptual Analysis: An Analysis of Conceptual Analysis in Philosophy of Medicine." *Theoretical Medicine and Bioethics* 34 (4): 309–325.

Lewis, David. 1994. "Reduction of Mind." In *Companion to the Philosophy of Mind*, edited by Samuel Guttenplan, 412–431. Oxford: Blackwell.

Matthews, Eric. 2009. "Against Definition." *Philosophy, Psychiatry, and Philosophy* 16 (1): 53–57.

Millikan, Ruth G. 1984. *Language, Thought and Other Biological Categories: New Foundations for Realism*. Cambridge, MA: MIT Press.

Morse, Stephen J. 2011. "Mental Disorder and Criminal Law." *The Journal of Criminal Law and Criminology* 101 (3): 885–968.

Murphy, Dominic. 2006. *Psychiatry in the Scientific Image*. Cambridge, MA: MIT Press.

Nordby, Halvor. 2006. "The Analytic-Synthetic Distinction and Conceptual Analyses of Basic Health Concepts." *Medicine, Health Care and Philosophy* 9 (2): 169–180.

Plato. 1952. *Plato's Phaedrus*. Cambridge: Cambridge University Press.

Schwartz, Peter H. 2007. "Defining Dysfunction: Natural Selection, Design, and Drawing a Line." *Philosophy of Science* 74 (3): 364–385.

———. 2014. "Reframing the Disease Debate and Defending the Biostatistical Theory." *Journal of Medicine and Philosophy* 39: 572–589.

Strawson, Peter F. 1992. *Analysis and Metaphysics: An Introduction to Philosophy*. Oxford: Oxford University Press.

Szasz, Thomas S. 1960. "The Myth of Mental Illness." *American Psychologist* 15: 113–118.

———. 1961. *The Myth of Mental Illness: Foundations of a Theory of Personal Conduct*. New York: Hoeber-Harper.

———. 1971. "The Sane Slave." *American Journal of Psychotherapy* 25 (2): 228–239.

Tasca, Cecilia, Mariangela Rapetti, Mauro Giovanni Carta, and Bianca Fadda. 2012. "Women and Hysteria in the History of Mental Health." *Clinical Practice and Epidemiology in Mental Health* 8: 110–119.

Ursano, Robert J., Carl Bell, Spencer Eth, Matthew Friedman, Ann Norwood, Betty Pfefferbaum, J. D. Robert S. Pynoos, Douglas F. Zatzick, David M. Benedek, John S. McIntyre, et al. 2004. "Practice Guideline for the Treatment of Patients with Acute Stress Disorder and Posttraumatic Stress Disorder." *American Journal of Psychiatry*, 161 (11): 3–31.

Wakefield, Jerome C. 2013. "The DSM-5 Debate over the Bereavement Exclusion: Psychiatric Diagnosis and the Future of Empirically Supported Treatment." *Clinical Psychology Review* 33 (7): 825–845.

———. 2016. "Diagnostic Issues and Controversies in DSM-5: Return of the False Positives Problem." *Annual Review of Clinical Psychology* 12: 105–132.

Watson, Gary. 2004. *Agency and Answerability: Selected Essays*. Oxford: Oxford University Press.

Wilkinson, Stephen. 2000. "Is 'Normal Grief' a Mental Disorder?" *The Philosophical Quarterly* 50 (200): 290–304.

World Health Organization (WHO) (ed.). 2019. *International Classification of Diseases 11ᵗʰ Edition (ICD-11)*. Geneva: World Health Organization.

2 Harm Views and Action Views

In Chapter 1, I have elaborated on the method of explication. I now move on to discussing the major prevalent views of the concept MENTAL DISORDER. In this chapter, I focus on Harm Views and Action Views.

Proponents of Harm Views typically hold that, for an individual S to have a mental disorder, it is necessary that S be in a mental condition that is *harmful* to S. Proponents of this view are, for instance, Danner Clouser, Charles Culver, and Bernard Gert (1981), Lawrie Reznek (1987, 1991), and Rachel Cooper (2005, 2007).[1] According to Harm Views, there is no such thing as a harmless disorder. Proponents of Harm Views agree that the presence of harm is not sufficient for having a disorder. There are many conditions that are harmful to S but that are not considered disorders (for example, unkemptness, forgetfulness, and recklessness). That said, proponents of Harm Views disagree on which further conditions are necessary to demarcate pathological from non-pathological harmful conditions. In this chapter, I discuss those Harm Views that put forward further conditions without referring to biological functions.

Proponents of Action Views (see Fulford 1989 and Nordenfelt 1995) have in common that they take health to consist in a set of abilities to act, and they take a disorder to be a kind of "failure of action" or impairment of the ability to φ (where φ is an action). As in Harm Views, proponents of Action Views take ascriptions of health and disorder to apply primarily to individuals as a whole, and only derivatively to their component parts. More specifically, their views imply that only agents can be subjected to disorders. Variations of Action Views differ with regard to the types of agentive abilities that are relevant for health.

This chapter is structured as follows. In Sections 2.1, 2.2, and 2.3, I discuss the Harm Views. In Sections 2.4 and 2.5, I discuss the Action Views. In Section 2.6, I evaluate the Harm Views and Action Views in light of the adequacy conditions outlined in Section 1.3.

DOI: 10.4324/9781003367840-3

2.1 Gert, Culver, and Clouser

Gert, Culver, and Clouser (GCC) define MALADY (in my terminology: DIS-ORDER) as follows:

> An individual has a malady if and only if she (he) has a condition, other than her (his) rational beliefs or desires, such that she (he) is suffering, or is at significantly increased risk of suffering, a nontrivial *harm* or evil (death, pain, disability, loss of freedom, or loss of pleasure) in the absence of a *distinct sustaining cause*.
>
> (2006, 142 f., my emphasis)

To define MENTAL DISORDER, we need simply to change "condition" to "mental condition." According to GCC (2006, 141), a distinct sustaining cause is an event that has an effect and whose removal results in the removal of the effect. For illustration, consider strangulation. An individual's condition under strangulation is not a disorder as long as stopping the strangulation also stops its effects.

GCC characterize HARM by listing different types of harms: death, pain, disability or loss of ability, loss of freedom, and loss of pleasure.[2] What do these phenomena have in common that makes their status as harms intelligible? GCC's answer is that

> no one wants them. In fact, everyone wants to avoid them. At least all individuals acting rationally want to avoid them unless they have an adequate reason not to.
>
> (2006, 136)

This characterization allows for two different readings. Something could be a harm because (a) every individual *de facto* wants to avoid it or (b) every individual acting rationally would want to avoid it unless they had an adequate reason not to. The first claim is an empirical one. We could test it by conducting a cross-cultural study, perhaps. The second claim is one about what a fully rational individual would (not) want to do.

Gert settles on the second reading, according to which harm "is best defined as that which all rational persons avoid unless they have an adequate reason not to" (2005, 91). On Gert's view, an "objectively adequate reason is an objective reason, that is, a fact that can make the particular otherwise objectively irrational action rational" (2005, 31, italics removed). Gert defines an irrational action as follows:

> A person correctly appraises an action as irrational when she correctly believes (1) it will cause, or significantly increase the probability of, the agent's

suffering (avoidable) death, pain, disability, loss of freedom, or loss of pleasure, and (2) there is no objectively adequate reason for the action.

(2005, 31, italics removed)

Let me now discuss three problems with GCC's view.

1 *Circularity*. Gert's definition of HARM is circular in an uninformative
way. To see why, let me reconstruct Gert's (2005) definitions more
formally:

1 φ-ing is a harm if and only if an individual S acting rationally would
never (want to) φ unless S had an adequate reason to φ.
2 An adequate reason to φ makes an irrational φ-ing rational.
3 A rational φ-ing is a φ-ing that is not irrational.
4 An irrational φ-ing is a φ-ing for which there is no adequate reason.
5 A rational φ-ing is a φ-ing for which there is an adequate reason
(from 3 and 4).
6 A rational φ-ing is a φ-ing for which there is a fact that makes an irrational φ-ing rational (from 2 and 5).

Thus, it turns out that φ-ing is a harm if and only if an individual S acting rationally would never (want to) φ unless there is a fact that makes
φ-ing rational. This definition is circular in an uninformative way because it leaves open the question of *when* a fact makes φ-ing rational.
In light of this, it is hard to see how a list of harms could be deduced
from it.

2 *Controversial List*. Lacking a satisfying definition of HARM would not
be problematic if GCC's list were uncontroversial. But it is not. Take,
for instance, Epicurus' (1966) argument against death being a harm.
Death is nothing to us because when we are, death is not; and when
death is, we are not. Although Epicurus' argument is somewhat unclear,
the point seems to be that neither being dead nor any posthumous event
for that matter can harm us. Either we are alive or we are dead, but,
when we are dead, nothing can affect us in a way that is bad for us (or
presumably good for us either). One might think that the process of dying can harm us, but only while it is occurring.

There are also other types of putative harms. Poverty, violence, and
loneliness are things that individuals (when acting rationally) generally
want to avoid (unless they have an adequate reason not to). So, why are
these not on GCC's list? Perhaps, because they are not *medically relevant* harms. But then, what makes a harm a medically relevant one?
These considerations suggest that GCC's "Objective List Theory" of
harm needs to be supported by further arguments.

3 *Extensional Inadequacy*. GCC's view of (MENTAL) DISORDER is overinclusive. As Boorse (2011, 53) points out, it seems to include menstruation, pregnancy, menopause, teething, and aging, which should clearly not count as disorders. Within the mental realm, conditions such as typical grief or lovesickness would count as mental disorders. This is because, typically, the lovesick and the individual in grief are suffering in the absence of a distinct sustaining cause. But typical grief and lovesickness should clearly not count as mental disorders.[3]

2.2 Reznek

Reznek defines PATHOLOGICAL CONDITION (in my terminology: DISORDER) as follows:

A has a pathological condition C if and only if A is an abnormal bodily/mental condition which requires medical intervention and for which medical intervention is appropriate, and which harms standard members of A's species in standard circumstances.

(1987, 167)

According to Reznek, "X does A some harm if and only if X makes A less able to lead a good or worthwhile life" (1987, 153) and our welfare "consists in the satisfaction of worthwhile desires and the enjoyment of worthwhile pleasures" (1987, 151).

Reznek holds that "normality" cannot be understood in a statistical sense because whole populations can suffer from disorders (for example, Ebola virus disease can become epidemic). Disorders can be statistically normal, while what is statistically abnormal (for instance, an ultramarathon runner's stamina) need not be pathological. On Reznek's view, we "choose one norm rather than another because we wish to create certain priorities in dealing with all those conditions that we would be better off without" (1987, 94). Reznek defends this claim by means of the example of aging:

If we discovered a drug that enabled us to live healthy lives to 200-years-old, would we not come to view the drug as vitamin F, and regard our present ageing process as abnormal and as a vitamin-deficiency disease?

(1987, 97)

The view that Reznek proposes seems to be the following: from a set of conditions that we would be better off without, we *choose* those conditions that should count as abnormal, and these will be the ones that we are (likely) able to treat medically. To talk about choice in this context is, however, misleading. It suggests decisionism about abnormality: what counts as abnormal is based on nothing more than the fact that we choose to count it as abnormal. But, even on Reznek's view, we do not simply choose the relevant conditions at will. We do so for a reason. For Reznek, abnormal harms are those that we are likely able to treat medically. To avoid misunderstandings, we should then avoid talking of choice in this context.

On Reznek's view, there is a strong link between having a disorder and requiring medical treatment. On his view, "judging that some condition is a disease commits one to stamping it out. And judging that a condition is not a disease commits one to preventing its medical treatment" (1987, 167). Thus, for Reznek, having a disorder gives the affected individual a decisive reason for medical treatment rather than a *pro tanto* reason. Moreover, it is not merely unnecessary to treat non-pathological conditions. Rather, non-pathological conditions should not be treated medically.

Reznek (1987) argues that being in a condition that requires medical treatment is a necessary condition for having a disorder. He does so by pointing out that there are various harmful conditions (for example, starvation or freezing) that we do not consider pathological, presumably because they can be removed through non-medical means (by eating or by wearing thermal clothing). In contrast, hypothermia is considered pathological because it requires medical treatment. On Reznek's view, medical treatment must also be "appropriate" (1987, 167). Even if we discovered that all people who have criminal records can be treated by some drug, we might decline to use it if we believe that it is up to each individual to choose whether to act criminally or not.

Let me now discuss five problems with Reznek's view.

1 *Abnormality.* The abnormality condition is redundant because abnormal conditions turn out to be just harmful conditions that can likely be medically treated (see Nordenfelt 2001, Boorse 2011, 2021 for similar objections). According to Reznek, what is abnormal is nothing more than what we choose to be abnormal, and what we choose to be abnormal is that which is likely medically treatable.

2 *Medical Treatability.* To be likely medically treatable is not a necessary condition for having a disorder. Boorse's (2011, 51) counterexamples are heat exhaustion and altitude sickness. These conditions are clearly pathological, but they are not likely medically treatable. Although it is possible to increase our tolerance for heat and altitude to some degree, it is not possible to extend it *ad infinitum*. An organism's bodily constitution limits its ability to deal with heat and high altitude.

3 *Back-to-Front.* Reznek's medical treatment claim gets things back-to-front. Contra Reznek, I would argue that disorders are not abnormal

conditions because they are likely medically treatable. If anything, we medically treat them because they are abnormal. Reznek (1987, 167) claims that MEDICAL TREATMENT can be defined only extensionally: medical treatments are drugs, surgery, and so on. Further types of treatments he mentions include psychoanalysis, behavior therapy, and cognitive therapy. However, the fact that Reznek uses the expression "and so on" suggests that there is something that all these types of treatments have in common. Spelled out, "and so on" means "and other things similar to those I have mentioned." But, in what respect are additional things similar to those already included in the set? It seems that everything that has a significant and measurable effect on ameliorating a disorder qualifies as a candidate for medical treatment. If prayer had significant measurable effects on ameliorating disorders, then we could consider it medical treatment. This suggests that the difference between MEDICAL TREAT-MENT and NON-MEDICAL TREATMENT depends on the concept DISORDER. Such a view has some intuitive appeal. Drinking water is not a medical treatment when one is healthy, but it is when one is dehydrated.

4 *Treatment Requirement.* The conceptual link between DISORDER and MEDICAL TREATMENT is not as tight as Reznek takes it to be. Having a disorder only provides the affected individual with a *pro tanto* reason to seek medical treatment. All things considered they may have sufficient reason not to treat it. In addition, it is conceptually possible that there are disorders that are impossible to treat.

5 *Extensional Inadequacy.* Given the aforementioned, Reznek's view seems to reduce to the claim that disorders are harmful conditions (in the sense that they are less able to satisfy worthwhile desires and enjoy worthwhile pleasures). But, this view of DISORDER presents another problem. There are various conditions that make the affected individuals less able to satisfy worthwhile desires and enjoy worthwhile pleasures that are not necessarily disorders. These include forgetfulness, recklessness, irritability, and so on. According to Cooper (2007, 37), being ugly or stupid makes an individual more worse off than putative disorders such as athlete's foot or eczema. Nevertheless, we normally consider athlete's foot and eczema to be disorders, while we do not normally consider ugliness and stupidity to be disorders. Further examples are illiteracy, having an incomprehensible accent, and vices such as laziness.[4]

2.3 Cooper

Cooper develops a variation of Reznek's view. According to Cooper (2002, 271, 2005, 22 ff.), an individual S has a disease (in my terminology: DIS-ORDER) if and only if S's condition is (1) a bad thing for S to have, (2) S is unlucky to have it, and (3) it is potentially medically treatable. I will elaborate on each of these conditions in turn.

1 *Badness.* Cooper discusses the following three "ways of determining" what is good for an individual:

> [1] At one end of the scale lie methods that rely on asking actual people what they want. [2] At the other end of the scale lie methods that claim that something is good for an individual if it helps that individual to meet some ideal standard of human flourishing. [3] In between these two extremes lie methods that claim that something is good for an individual if that individual would judge it to be good in ideal circumstances, for example if they had all the information, and were calmer and wiser than they probably are.
>
> (2005, 24)

It is not clear whether these "ways of determining" are best understood as epistemic criteria for finding out what is good for an individual or as necessary conditions for something to be good for an individual. Cooper, though, refutes all three such ways. (1) Asking people what they want is problematic because "people often do not know what is in their best interest" (2002, 273). (2) Referring to an ideal of human flourishing is "disturbingly anti-naturalistic," and "it is not at all clear how the ideal standards are fixed, nor is it clear how we can find out about them" (2005, 25). (3) Judgments about ideal circumstances bear epistemic problems: "I know what I actually value, but how can I know what I'd value if I were more knowledgeable and wiser than I actually am?" (2005, 25). Cooper concludes that we should "just make use of our everyday intuitions concerning the badness of various conditions" (2002, 274).

On closer inspection, it appears that, on Cooper's view, for an individual's condition to be good for them to have, is for it to be in their *best interest*. And what *is* in an individual's best interest is not constituted by what they *say* is in their best interest, nor by what they say they want. Individuals may not know what is in their best interest because they may be falsely or insufficiently informed.

However, this view stands in tension with some of Cooper's other claims. According to Cooper (2005), a condition might be pathological for one individual but not for another. She argues as follows:

> The schizophrenic for whom it is a good thing to be schizophrenic is not diseased, while another for whom it is a bad thing is. Here I am suggesting that we should think about diseases in a way analogous to the way in which we think about weeds. A plant is only a weed if it is not wanted. Thus, a daisy can be a weed in one garden but a

flower in another, depending on whether or not it is a good thing in a particular garden.

(2005, 26)

A weed is simply a plant that is unwanted by some individual or group in a particular context. The analogy suggests that whether a phenomenon such as schizophrenia is a type of disorder is determined by whether it is wanted by the affected individual. To strengthen this claim, Cooper (2002, 275) points out that sterility is a disorder if unchosen but not if it is the result of voluntary sterilization. Here, Cooper equates what is good with what is wanted. Thus, it appears that Cooper's view on what constitutes a disorder is inconsistent.

2 *Unluckiness*. According to Cooper, an individual is unlucky if, and only if they "could reasonably have hoped to have been otherwise" (2005, 30). That is, "there must be a good number of possible worlds consistent with the laws of human biology where people like [them] are in a better state" (2005, 30). What counts is the layperson's judgment of whether one is "roughly, worse off than the majority of humans of the same sex and age" (2002, 276) and not the judgment of a scientist. Human biology requires teething, but it does not require blindness.

3 *Medical Treatability*. According to Cooper, bad but unlucky conditions that are easily treatable by non-medical methods (her examples are obesity or a bad haircut) are not diseases. Only conditions that are potentially medically treatable are diseases. Cooper claims that there is "no way of distinguishing some medical interventions from some non-medical interventions in terms of what is actually done" (2002, 278). Instead, she proposes adopting the following approach. Medical interventions are interventions practiced by doctors and other medical personnel. Who counts as "doctors and other medical personnel" should be decided by adopting a "sociological approach" (Cooper 2002, 278). Moreover, conditions are potentially medically treatable if "there is reasonable hope that a medical treatment might become available in the future" (Cooper 2002, 277).

Let me now discuss two problems with Cooper's view.

1 *Extensional Inadequacy*. Cooper's conception is extensionally inadequate because it is overinclusive. Consider Sage, an individual with extraordinarily high intellectual abilities. Sage suffers from their condition of being a genius because they cannot bear the stupidity of their peers and they are socially isolated owing to their high intelligence. Furthermore, Sage feels pressured to achieve something extraordinary with their intellectual abilities. They really do not want to be so

intelligent. Sage is also unlucky to have these abilities because there are a good number of possible worlds consistent with the laws of human biology where they are less intelligent than they are in this world. There are, though, various psychoactive drugs that might help Sage overcome their condition. On Cooper's view, Sage's case is an instance of DISORDER. But this seems *prima facie* absurd. We would not normally consider Sage's unhappiness to be a disorder.

Cooper could attempt to refute this objection by replying that Sage's condition of being a genius is not bad for them. In fact, Cooper (2002, 272) explicitly denies that geniuses have a disorder; they are not in a bad condition, but merely biologically different. However, if being a genius is never bad, then "being bad" cannot be synonymous with "being unwanted" because clearly, an individual can want to be less intelligent. But, then, analogizing DISORDER to WEED is problematic. Cooper could possibly retreat to the view that it is an individual's best interests that counts and not what they want. But this does not solve the problem either. It is not too far-fetched to believe that it might be in Sage's best interest for them to be less intelligent.

Even if we rely on everyday intuitions about which types of conditions are bad, Cooper's conception is overinclusive. The list of counterexamples includes being ugly, unintelligent, boring, or unpleasant, and so on. These all count as disorders on Cooper's view. But, as we have seen, this is not necessarily the case. This suggests that being biologically unlucky must be distinguished from having a disorder. Although someone with a disorder is in some sense biologically unlucky, not everyone who is biologically unlucky has a disorder in virtue thereof.

2 *Conceptual Unclarity*. Cooper's claim that a condition must be potentially medically treatable suffers from conceptual problems. What exactly does it mean to determine who counts as doctors and medical personnel on a "sociological approach"? If a layperson performs an emergency operation to save someone's life, are they not then performing a medical intervention? And, what exactly can we "reasonably hope for"? Is it reasonable to hope for a medical treatment for influenza or cancer? It is highly counterintuitive to categorize some condition as a disease depending on whether or not that condition can be treated. It is like saying that a system can be broken only if there is a chance that it might be repaired.

2.4 Fulford

Fulford identifies three concepts as counterparts to HEALTH: ILLNESS, DISEASE, and DYSFUNCTION. For Fulford, these concepts are not identical, although they are closely related (1989, 27 f.). For instance, an individual with controlled diabetes or asymptomatic cancer has a disease, but they are not ill. An individual suffering from a migraine is ill but does not have a disease. MIGRAINE is not defined as a dysfunction, but by the fact that an individual suffers a certain type of headache. Headache is a symptom that is associated with many types of diseases or dysfunctions.

According to Fulford (1989, 30), ILLNESS provides the most general understanding of HEALTH-related concepts (which then corresponds to DISORDER in my terminology). On Fulford's view, this is the primary concept from which all others can be derived. Fulford makes two points to motivate his view. First, he claims that the expression "an individual is ill" expresses a negative value judgment: the judgment "[s]omething with that individual is wrong" (1989, 30).[5] In contrast, the expression "[a]n individual has a disease" expresses the judgment "[t]his with that individual is wrong" (1989, 30). For Fulford, ILLNESS is more general than DISEASE because ascriptions of disease specify *what* is wrong with an individual.

Second, Fulford argues that we ascribe illnesses to individuals as a whole, but we ascribe dysfunctions to parts of bodies or parts of organisms (1989, 32). If DYSFUNCTION were the primary concept, then the claim "an individual is ill" would translate to "an individual is not functioning properly." But this, argues Fulford, is not how we speak. People fall ill, but it is their bodies (or parts of their bodies) that fail to function properly. Fulford concludes that ILLNESS is therefore more general than DYSFUNCTION.

In light of this, the challenge for a conceptual analysis consists in spelling out the exact sense in which an illness entails that something is wrong with an individual. To analyze ILLNESS, Fulford asks the following. In the same way that a bodily dysfunction stands in relation to its proper functioning, what does an individual's illness stand in relation to? Fulford claims that the answer is *ordinary action*. While a dysfunction is a failure of proper functioning of some part of an organism, an "illness [has] its origins in the experience of a particular kind of action failure—failure of what is here called 'ordinary' doing in the apparent absence of obstruction and/or opposition" (Fulford 1989, 109).[6] Thus, when it comes to illness, something is wrong when an affected individual fails to perform some ordinary action(s).

Fulford's characterization of what ordinary actions are, however, is unspecific. According to Fulford (1989, 116), they are actions that are performed in the "everyday way in which people do things," or citing John L. Austin, they are actions that we "just get on and do." Furthermore,

[t]o say, with Austin, that in doing something one "just gets on and does it", is really to say no more than that one is not, at the time, reflecting on one's intentions, or indeed on any other element of the full sense of "do".
(Fulford 1989, 117)

Examples of ordinary actions are everyday routines like getting out of bed, making coffee, brushing one's teeth, putting on clothes, and so on. Ordinary actions can also be actions performed without much attention (or without prior intention or planning). These include scratching one's nose, walking, thinking, and talking. It follows that ordinary action can be understood in, at least, two senses: (a) generally, as any type of action that could be performed without much attention or (b) narrowly, as everyday actions or routines.

What is it to *fail* to perform an ordinary action? Failing to φ is not the same as not φ-ing. My not brushing my teeth counts as a failure only if I intended to brush my teeth. Otherwise, I simply did not do it. More generally, an agent fails to φ if they intend to φ, but do not φ. Thus, an individual fails to perform an ordinary action if they intend to φ (where φ is an ordinary action) but do not φ.

According to Fulford, there are many kinds of disease, but they are all defined in relation to ILLNESS. Sometimes "disease" means "illnesses that are widely considered as such;" at other times, it means "conditions that are causally or statistically associated with illnesses that are widely considered as such" (Fulford 1989, 59). Thus, either (a) DISEASE is a subcategory of ILLNESS or (b) the conditions that fall under DISEASE are causes of or correlated with conditions that fall under ILLNESS. Although Fulford claims that DYSFUNCTION can be derived from ILLNESS, he does not provide a definition or characterization of it.

Fulford recognizes that many illnesses are characterized by pain and other negative sensations (for example, nausea or itchiness) that are ostensibly not failures of ordinary action. He claims nonetheless that he can account for these cases in terms of failures of action. He argues that a healthy individual can normally withdraw from pain and negative sensations (for example, by removing their hand from a hot stove). But, in illness, one experiences "pain from which one is unable to withdraw in the (perceived) absence of obstruction and/or opposition" (Fulford 1989, 138). Pain and negative sensations are illnesses only if the affected individual is unable to stop them (but would be able to do so under normal conditions).

Let me now discuss seven problems with Fulford's view.

1 *Not Sufficient*. Failure of ordinary action (in both senses) is not sufficient for having an illness. A grandparent of mine regularly fails to open bottles because they are not strong enough. Lazy people may regularly fail to wash the dishes. Menstrual pain may lead to failure of ordinary action. But in none of these cases is the individual necessarily ill.

2 *Not Necessary*. Failure of ordinary action is not necessary for having a disorder (neither a bodily nor a mental disorder). Cooper (2007, 35)

argues that Fulford cannot account for disfiguring conditions and "pathological sensations" (for example, distortions of the visual field or sensations of depersonalizations). Being disfigured need not interfere with an individual's ability to perform ordinary actions, nor is it characterized by an unpleasant sensation from which they would normally withdraw. Moreover, many pathological sensations are not sensations that we can normally stop. In fact, they are sensations that we normally do not experience at all. Hence, it makes no sense to claim that a lack of ability to withdraw from such sensations is a failure of something that we can normally do.

Boorse (2011, 40) argues that Fulford's view cannot account for psychosis, which is one of the paradigmatic examples of a mental disorder. Even if psychosis were defined in terms of practical irrationality with respect to ordinary actions, this would not imply that irrational ordinary action is not an action. If individuals with psychosis have the ability to perform an irrational ordinary action, then they obviously have the ability to perform a general ordinary action (albeit an irrational one). Hence, they do not lack the ability to perform an ordinary action.

Fulford could reply as follows. It is possible for an individual to lack the ability to φ_1 without (a) lacking the ability to φ_2 or (b) lacking the ability to φ altogether. An individual with a broken arm may lack the ability to raise their arm, but they clearly do not thereby lack the ability to walk, talk, or perform most other actions that they can usually perform. Hence, it is consistent to claim that an individual with psychosis lacks the ability to perform certain types of actions without being committed to the claim that they lack the ability to perform other types of actions or lack the ability to act altogether.

In any case, Fulford's view is inadequate with respect to mental disorders. It is possible for an individual to have a major depressive disorder, for example, without failing to perform any ordinary action they intend to perform. Although individuals with a major depressive disorder are often seriously impaired in their ability to perform certain types of ordinary actions (for example, getting out of bed or maintaining an everyday routine), such impairments are not necessary. Such individuals may be able to function socially, but still be depressed. Moreover, in some cases of mental disorder (for example, a manic episode of bipolar disorder), an individual might even be able to perform ordinary actions better than they normally would (see Boorse 2011, 40).

3 *Inconsistency.* Fulford's view of the relationship between DISEASE and ILLNESS is inconsistent. Fulford claims that not all diseases are illnesses. But he also claims that ILLNESS is more general than DISEASE (in that the former implies *that* something is wrong with an individual, while the

latter describes *what* is wrong with an individual). However, if this were true, then all diseases are necessarily illnesses because any specification of what is wrong with an individual presupposes that something is wrong with them.

4 *Illness versus Disease.* Even if DISEASE is not a subcategory of ILLNESS, but merely conditions that cause or correlate with conditions falling under ILLNESS, ILLNESS is too narrow to define DISEASE. Boorse (2014, 44) mentions a cataract that can cause blindness and the degeneration of hair cells in the inner ear that can cause deafness. Although blindness and deafness are clearly diseases (given current medical practice), neither is an illness. In fact, Boorse (2011) argues that most conditions treated by medical specialties (for example, ophthalmology, otolaryngology, dermatology) are neither illnesses nor do they cause or correlate with illnesses.

5 *Dysfunction versus Illness.* Fulford does not show how DYSFUNCTION can be derived from ILLNESS. In fact, it is unlikely that one can derive the former from the latter on the assumption that illness is a failure of ordinary action. Because actions require an agent, actions and failures of actions can be ascribed only to agents. Individuals are agents, but parts of an individual's body are not. Hence, illness cannot be ascribed to parts of an individual's body. However, as Fulford acknowledges, dysfunctions are ascribed to parts of an individual's body. Thus, the only way an individual's failure to act could enter a definition of DYS-FUNCTION is by stating that something is a dysfunction only if it causes or correlates with a failure of action. But, then again, one could object that not all dysfunctions have effects on a personal level.

6 *Semantics versus Ontology.* The fact that dysfunctions are ascribed to parts of the body and illness to individuals does not support the conclusion that ILLNESS is primary to DYSFUNCTION. Some bodily parts to which dysfunctions are ascribed are parts of an individual's body to which illnesses are ascribed. But this does not show that the concept DYS-FUNCTION is a subcategory of the concept ILLNESS. A semantic relation between the concepts DYSFUNCTION and ILLNESS does not follow from the ontological parts-whole relation between organs and organisms.

7 *Personal and Sub-personal "Functioning."* Fulford's claim that we do not make statements like "an individual is not functioning properly" is only partly true. We make statements like "an individual is not functioning well in social contexts." Thus, we sometimes state that individuals as a whole are functioning better or worse. This suggests that we naturally distinguish between two senses of "functioning": one on a personal level and one on a sub-personal level.

2.5 Nordenfelt

Nordenfelt begins his analysis of HEALTH with the following intuition:

> A person is healthy if he feels well and can function in his social context. [...] We intuitively connect health with well-being and ability, and illness with suffering and disability, and view these features as their *essential* characteristics.
>
> (1995, 37)

Nordenfelt also assumes that there is a conceptual relation between SUFFERING and DISABILITY:

> Being in great pain, for instance, partly *means* that one is disabled. Some degree of disability is here a necessary condition for the presence of pain, so that if a person's ability is not affected, he can be said not to be in great pain.
>
> (1995, 35)

Hence, for Nordenfelt, an individual can have a disability without suffering, but not the other way around. When analyzing HEALTH, DISABILITY is taken to be the central concept.

Moreover, according to Nordenfelt, for an agent A to be healthy is for A to have the ability to *achieve their vital goals*:

> A is healthy if, and only if, A has the second-order ability, given standard circumstances, to realize all the goals necessary for his minimal happiness.
>
> (1995, 79)

Nordenfelt's "Welfare View" of health is thus based on three concepts: ACTION, ABILITY, and VITAL GOAL. I will elaborate on each of these concepts in turn.

1 *Action.* Nordenfelt considers actions to be a subclass of bodily movements, namely those that are caused by an intention: "To shake one's hand or to nod one's head is an action only if the agent intends to do so" (1995, 37). For Nordenfelt, stating that an individual subjected to illness "cannot" perform certain actions can have different meanings. Two of these are important for an analysis of HEALTH. That an individual "cannot" φ can mean (1) that they do not have the *ability* to φ or (2) that they do not have the *opportunity* to φ. "I cannot swim," for

instance, could mean that I lack the ability to swim (I have never learned to do so) or that I do not have the opportunity to exercise my ability to swim (I am not close to swimmable water). To have what Nordenfelt (1995) calls the "practical possibility" to φ, both are required: the ability and the opportunity to φ. However, Nordenfelt does not provide a definition of ABILITY. Instead, he claims that we can test whether it is practically possible for an agent A to φ (where φ is an action) by letting A try to φ. If A attempts to φ and succeeds, then it is practically possible for A to φ (Nordenfelt 1995, 42).

2 *Ability.* Nordenfelt distinguishes between first-order and second-order abilities. He characterizes second-order abilities as follows:

> A has a second-order ability with regard to an action F, if and only if, A has the first-order ability to pursue a training-program after the completion of which A will have the first-order ability to do F.
>
> (1995, 50)

In other words, a second-order ability to φ is the ability to *learn* the ability to φ. According to Nordenfelt, not having a first-order ability is not sufficient for having an illness. His example is "a newcomer to Sweden who has problems taking care of himself" (1995, 51). According to Nordenfelt, the newcomer is ill only if he does "not have the second-order ability to manage his living in the new environment" (1995, 51).

3 *Vital Goal.* Nordenfelt (1995, 55) maintains that not all of our second-order abilities are relevant for an analysis of HEALTH, but rather only those that aid us in achieving our vital goals. On this view, an individual's vital goals are identical neither to humans' basic needs for survival nor with their self-chosen goals. Basic needs for survival are too narrow to determine the vital goals relevant for health because many unhealthy people can fulfill their basic needs for survival. Self-chosen goals are too wide to determine the vital goals relevant for health because they would render, for example, highly ambitious people unhealthy.

Nordenfelt proposes that the "vital goals of man are those whose fulfillment is necessary and jointly sufficient for a minimal degree of welfare, i.e. happiness" (1995, 78). Happiness, in turn, is an emotion often experienced when some of our needs or goals are fulfilled (Nordenfelt 1995, 82). For Nordenfelt, being happy about surviving is not sufficient to constitute minimal happiness. He puts it as follows:

> "Real" happiness presupposes a minimum of complexity and subtlety. A person who fulfills a very small and primitive set of goals does not

fulfill the requirements of minimal *human* welfare, minimal human happiness. Thus, if his abilities do not supersede the ability to fulfill his primitive goals, then he cannot be healthy.

(1995, 79)

So, it is roughly the fulfillment of specifically human needs or goals that is relevant for health and not merely the fulfillment of those needs that human beings share with other living things (for example, the need for food). Besides having food, Nordenfelt (1995, 60 ff.) claims that the following are basic human needs or goals: having a sheltered home, some economic security, some intellectual pleasures, and some pleasures of bodily locomotion.

Nordenfelt concedes that, on this conception of HEALTH, there could be medical and non-medical illnesses. He does not elaborate on this distinction, but merely points out certain examples. He takes medical illnesses to be what GCC call "maladies," that is, diseases, injuries, impairments, and defects. Although maladies do not always cause illnesses, the two phenomena are related in important ways. For Nordenfelt (1995, 105 ff.), a disease is an internal process that is likely to cause illness in a given environment.

Let me discuss three problems with Nordenfelt's view.

1 *Extensional Inadequacy.* Nordenfelt's claim that a disorder consists in a lack of the second-order ability to achieve some of one's vital goals is implausible. If a second-order ability to φ is the ability to learn the ability to φ, then not having a second-order ability is not necessary for having a disorder. Obviously, people can recover from having a mental disorder (for example, an addictive or anxiety disorder). Hence, they have the second-order ability to learn the relevant ability to achieve some of their vital goals.

Furthermore, as Boorse (2011, 44) points out, not all disorders involve failures or impairments of actions, and *a fortiori*, they do not involve failures of actions to achieve some of one's vital goals. Disfiguring conditions, pathological sensations, skin conditions, or specific phobias (for example, arachnophobia) need not affect an individual's abilities to achieve their vital goals. They may be obstacles, but they are not insurmountable ones.

Even more, Boorse argues that Nordenfelt's conception diverges sharply from medical judgments "by allowing a person with a systemic disease not to be ill, while a person frustrated by a normal physical condition may be seriously ill" (2011, 42). Consider a philosopher who has finally gotten tenure at their favorite university (which was one of their vital goals). However, at the same time, they suffer from diabetes and a panic disorder. They may be happier now that they have tenure than they would have been with neither the disorders nor the professional success. Yet, despite their being this happy, we should not deny that they are suffering from a disease or illness. However, such a denial seems to be exactly what Nordenfelt's view yields. On Nordenfelt's view, we would have to deny the philosopher's illness because their ability to achieve their vital goals allows them to achieve great happiness despite what we would normally call serious disorders.

Nordenfelt might reply that it is not the self-chosen goals that are relevant to the assessment of health but rather more modest goals such as having a sheltered home, some economic security, and so on. Yet, even then, Nordenfelt is committed to the view that the philosopher is healthy because they have these vital goals despite their panic disorder and diabetes.

2 *Conceptual Unclarity.* Examples like those just mentioned show that Nordenfelt's conception of VITAL GOAL is underdeveloped. It seems plausible to assume that having a sheltered home qualifies as a vital goal, but that getting tenure does not. But why? Without further elaboration, the list of vital goals seems arbitrary and *ad hoc*. This leads Thomas Schramme to claim that Nordenfelt has a stipulated definition of HEALTH, one that promotes the "medicalization of all kinds of problems in life" (2007, 15).

2.6 Harm Views and Action Views Evaluated

In this section, I will evaluate the discussed Harm Views and Action Views in light of the adequacy conditions outlined in Section 1.3.

2.6.1 Mental Disorder versus Mental Health

In the previous sections, I have argued that the Harm Views and Action Views are extensionally inadequate with respect to some clear cases of mental health and disorder. More specifically, the presence of harm is not sufficient for having a mental disorder, and the conditions mentioned in Action Views are neither necessary nor sufficient for having a mental disorder. Let me summarize and generalize the main points.

I begin with the Harm Views. That a mental condition is harmful to the affected individual is not sufficient for having a mental disorder. Examples of mental conditions that are harmful to the affected individuals, but not necessarily pathological, include unkemptness, forgetfulness, recklessness, irascibility, timidity, shyness, and irresoluteness. Even when introducing further conditions—distinct sustaining cause, potential medical treatability, bad luck—the scope of Harm Views is too wide. They include conditions that are clearly not disorders.

Moreover, none of the Harm Views can adequately explain why depression, for example, counts as a mental disorder while grief does not. In both depression and grief, the affected individual is harmed. However, grief has no distinct sustaining cause. On an *event* view of causation, an individual's dying process has an end: their death. But our grief typically sets in after the individual has died. On a *fact* view of causation, one could argue that the fact that one has suffered a loss is the cause of one's grief, and the cause of one's grief thus persists. Grief would then have a distinct sustaining cause. However, this view is implausible for independent reasons. If we regarded the fact that an individual has suffered a loss as the cause of their grief, then we can hardly explain why they ever stop grieving. Yet, individuals typically stop grieving after some time. Moreover (against Reznek and Cooper), grief might be medically treatable. If it is possible to treat anxiety, fear, and depression, then why should it not be possible to treat grief?

Conversely, depression might have a distinct sustaining cause (say, the continued intake of a hormone). And, even if it were not treatable, we would consider it a mental disorder (there are, after all, untreatable disorders). It is also implausible that there are "a good number of possible worlds consistent with the laws of human biology" (Cooper 2005, 30), where humans have the disposition to grieve but not to get depressed. Thus, it also does not make sense to believe that depression is an "unluckier" condition than grief, in Cooper's (2005) sense of the term.

Furthermore, an individual who has suffered the recent loss of a loved one would be better off, in some sense, by not grieving than by grieving (they would suffer less). Yet, it is not clear that they would be healthier. Typical grief is considered a healthy response to the recent loss of a loved one. Consider an individual who suffers the sudden loss of a spouse whom they valued highly and with whom they shared a long and happy life. It would be odd if they did not grieve at all when suffering such a loss (taking into account that there are culturally relative expressions of grief). We would suspect that either they did not value their spouse after all or that something has "gone awry" with their mental state (in a psychological or psychiatric sense).

I now turn to Action Views. A failure of ordinary action or an impaired ability to achieve one's vital goals is neither necessary nor sufficient for having a mental disorder. Consider a successful and happy philosopher who has no trouble performing their everyday routines but has arachnophobia or experiences manic episodes. Action Views would suggest that the philosopher does not have a mental disorder, although it is clearly possible that they do have one. Cases like these show that neither failure of ordinary action nor an impaired ability to achieve one's vital goals are necessary for having a mental disorder. These conditions are also not sufficient for having a mental disorder. Consider an individual who suffers from grief in response to the recent loss of a loved one or an individual who is in love but whose love is unrequited. They may have trouble sleeping, eating, and concentrating. Because of this, they may fail to perform some of their everyday routines and (temporarily) be impaired in their ability to achieve their vital goals or attain minimal happiness. Do they have a mental disorder? Maybe some of them do, but it is not necessary that all of them do.

That said, both Harm Views and Action Views do point to important aspects of mental disorders. Harm is *prima facie* a good candidate for accounting for some normative purposes (see Section 1.2) given the explicative project I am pursuing. And there seems to be something to the idea that disorders are connected in relevant ways to abilities. In Chapter 4, I shall present a view that incorporates both ideas.

2.6.2 Mental Disorder versus Bodily Disorder

Harm Views rarely discuss the distinction between mental disorders and bodily disorders. One option would be to argue that mental disorders are harmful mental conditions, whereas bodily disorders are harmful bodily conditions. One would then have to spell out what makes a condition a mental condition and how mental and bodily conditions relate to each other. Another option would be to distinguish between mental harm and bodily harm. Pain is often considered a bodily harm, whereas feelings of anxiety or depression are often considered mental harms.[7] But, this option is problematic because it is not clear what we could mean by "mental harm" if not "harmful mental condition." Semantically, it makes more sense to distinguish between "harmful mental conditions" and "harmful bodily conditions" (assuming that they are harmful in the same sense) than to claim that there are two senses of "harmful": a mental and a bodily one.

In any case, it is inadequate to explicate the distinction between mental disorders and bodily disorders in terms of harmful mental conditions *versus* harmful bodily conditions. Consider the following example. According to the *DSM-5* (APA 2013, 311), an individual experiences one or more somatic symptoms when suffering from somatic symptom disorder. These symptoms might include localized pain, fatigue, or even normal bodily sensations that are distressing or result in significant disruptions of daily life. If bodily disorders are harmful bodily conditions, and, if pain, fatigue, and bodily sensations are (merely) bodily conditions, then somatic symptom disorder should be considered a bodily disorder. However, it is not and should not be considered as such. It makes sense to distinguish somatic symptom disorders from bodily disorders because doing so gives *pro tanto* reasons for different types of treatments. We should not treat somatic symptom disorder in the same way as we treat (merely) bodily disorders, even if they are associated with the same symptoms.

Action Views also rarely discuss the distinction between mental and bodily disorders. According to Fulford, having an illness is failing to perform an ordinary action. On this view, one possible way to analyze the difference between MENTAL DISORDER and BODILY DISORDER is the following: BODILY DISORDER is a failure to perform an (ordinary) bodily action, whereas MENTAL DISORDER is a failure to perform an (ordinary) mental action. But this view is clearly false. Consider two individuals who miss the bus. One of them does so because of a broken leg and the other because of experiencing a panic attack. In both cases, the type of action they fail to perform is the same—namely, getting on a bus. But the former is clearly a case of bodily disorder, while the latter is clearly a case of mental disorder. Thus, the difference between MENTAL DISORDER and BODILY DISORDER cannot be analyzed by reference to the type of action that an individual fails to perform.

Nordenfelt's view is better off with respect to this distinction. A survey of the literature on abilities reveals that abilities are always possessed *in view of* certain facts (see Jaster 2020). Thus, one might suggest the following: whether an individual has a bodily disorder or a mental disorder depends on whether they are impaired in their ability to φ given their bodily constitution or their mental constitution. Applied to the previous example, this yields the following: the individual who fails to catch the bus because of experiencing a panic attack has a mental disorder because they are impaired in their ability to catch the bus in view of their mental constitution. The individual who fails to catch the bus because of a broken leg has a bodily disorder because they are impaired in the ability to catch the bus in view of their bodily constitution. Of course, this would only be the first step to clarifying the relation between MENTAL DISORDER and BODILY DISORDER. To develop a comprehensive view, one would have to say something about what makes a constitution a MENTAL or a BODILY one.

2.6.3 *Mental Disorder versus Deviance from Social, Legal, or Moral Norms*

Proponents of Harm Views have difficulties capturing and explaining the distinction between mental disorders and conditions that (merely) deviate from social, legal, or moral norms. Consider an individual suffering from self-neglect. They are clearly harmed by their condition, and it is possible that they violate certain social, legal, or moral standards as a result of their condition. But when and why is this condition *medically* relevant? Harm Views do not provide an answer to this question, but simply offer a list of what are taken to be medically relevant conditions.

One option for Harm Views to capture the distinction in question is to distinguish between *harm to oneself* and *harm to others*. Mental disorders will (only) involve harm to oneself and deviances from social, legal, or, moral norms will (only) involve harm to others. But this will not work. Again, an individual may suffer harm without having a mental disorder. Furthermore, harm to others is not necessary for social, legal, or moral deviance. It is possible to violate some of these by only harming oneself.

In contrast, proponents of Action Views do elaborate on the distinction between mental disorders and (mere) deviances from social, legal, or moral norms. Consider a case of neglect. A parent regularly fails to provide their 4-year-old child with food. This is clearly a case of an individual failing to perform some ordinary action: providing their child with food. In some cases (for example, food is available), this action violates certain social, legal, and moral norms. We rightly expect parents to take care of their children (unless they are excused from this duty for exceptional reasons). Furthermore, cases of neglect may be punishable by law. Section 171 of the German Criminal Code "Breach of duty of care or upbringing" states the following:

> Whoever grossly neglects their duty of care or upbringing towards a person under 16 years of age, thereby creating a danger that the physical or mental development of the person placed in their charge could be seriously damaged or that they will engage in crime or prostitution, incurs a penalty of imprisonment for a term not exceeding three years or a fine.
> (Federal Ministry of Justice and Consumer Protection, n.d.)

Cases like this show that Fulford's action view does not adequately demarcate mental disorders from cases of deviance from social, legal, or moral norms. If failure of ordinary action were sufficient, then there could not be cases in which there is both a failure of ordinary action and a violation of social, legal, or moral norms. But, of course, such cases are possible. Failure of ordinary action does not guarantee (a) the presence of a mental disorder (the parent could fail to feed their child without having a mental disorder) nor (b) that there is no violation of a social, legal, or moral norm if the individual who fails to perform an ordinary action has a mental disorder.

As before, Nordenfelt's view appears to be better off. There seems to be something to the idea that abilities can explain the distinction in question. This has to do with the fact that a lack or impairment of ability may sometimes excuse or exempt an individual from some of their actions. Our default view is that an adult is blameworthy when they are violating a social, legal, or moral norm unless (a) they have sufficient reason for such a violation, or (b) they have an excusing or exempting condition. In some cases, having a mental disorder of some kind is the excusing or exempting condition. Explicating MENTAL DISORDER in terms of (a lack of) abilities could provide the missing link that explains why having a mental disorder sometimes excuses or exempts an individual from certain violations of social, legal, or moral norms.

2.6.4 Normative Purposes

Harm Views can partly explain why having a mental disorder provides the affected individual with a *pro tanto* reason to seek psychiatric or psychotherapeutic treatment. All things being equal, harmless pathological conditions do not call for medical treatment, only harmful ones do. Generally, we value individuals' well-being, and any mental condition that is harmful to them is worthy of concern. However, harm itself cannot explain why having a mental disorder calls for psychiatric or psychotherapeutic attention rather than some other kind of attention. Harm can also explain some of the other normative consequences, but not all of them. To be harmed may be a sufficient reason for an individual to stay away from work, but it may not be sufficient to excuse moral or legal violations.

Action Views referring to abilities can, in some cases, explain why other people have a *pro tanto* reason to (a) (partly) excuse an individual with a mental disorder from certain actions, (b) release them from certain (social, legal, or moral) duties, or (c) offer them certain benefits. On an ability-based view of mental disorder, for instance, one might argue that, in some cases, having a manic episode excuses an individual from responsibility for some of their actions because they were in the relevant sense "not able to do otherwise." The challenge for such a view is to specify the exact sense in which an individual with a mental disorder is "not able to do otherwise." That said, an impairment of ability need not have any normative consequences. That an individual is not able to perform a certain type of action does not necessarily give them sufficient or decisive reason to do anything about it. I cannot do a handstand, for instance, but that does not give me sufficient or decisive reason to learn how to do one.

Notes

1 Other proponents of such a view are Engelhardt (1975), Culver and Gert (1982), Fulford (1989), Wakefield (1992), Thagard (1999), Hucklenbroich (2008), and Ereshefsky (2009).
2 In Clouser, Culver, and Gert (1981), they mention only death, pain, and disability as types of harms.
3 But couldn't GCC hold that the fact that a person is dead *is* a distinct sustaining cause of the other person's grief? They could, but this view would raise a different problem. On this view, grief could never be pathological. But this consequence should also be avoided. In some cases, grief can become pathological, see "persistent complex bereavement disorder" in the *DSM-5* (APA 2013).
4 This problem arises also for Aristotelian views of mental disorder (for such a view, see Megone 2000). Megone (2000) defines a flourishing life in a way that

is very close to Aristotle's original view. A flourishing life is a rational life: "the human function is [...] the life of the fully rational animal. Illness is any incapacitating failure to realize (actualize) this human function" (Megone 2000, 56). Here too, illiteracy and laziness turn out to be disorders.

5 This is why Fulford takes ILLNESS to be a value-laden concept. Because all other HEALTH-related concepts are derived from ILLNESS, they are then also value-laden.

6 This "apparent absence of obstruction and/or opposition" is similar to GCC's (2006) "distinct sustaining cause" (see Section 2.1).

7 See Section 5.5 for a further discussion of the mental/bodily distinction in philosophy and psychiatry.

References

American Psychiatric Association (APA). 2013. *Diagnostic and Statistical Manual of Mental Disorders: DSM-5*. Arlington: American Psychiatric Association.

Boorse, Christopher. 2011. "Concepts of Health and Disease." In *Philosophy of Medicine*, edited by Fred Gifford, 13–64. Munich: Elsevier.

———. 2014. "A Second Rebuttal on Health." *Journal of Medicine and Philosophy* 39 (6): 683–724.

———. 2021. "Reznek on Health." *Teorema* 40 (1): 23–65.

Clouser, K. Danner, Culver, Charles M., and Gert, Bernard. 1981. "Malady: A New Treatment of Disease." *The Hastings Center Report* 11 (3): 29–37.

Cooper, Rachel. 2002. "Disease." *Studies in History and Philosophy of Science* 33 (2): 263–282.

———. 2005. *Classifying Madness: A Philosophical Examination of the Diagnostic and Statistical Manual of Mental Disorders*. Dordrecht: Springer.

———. 2007. *Psychiatry and Philosophy of Science*. Durham: Acumen.

Culver, Charles M., and Bernard Gert. 1982. *Philosophy in Medicine. Conceptual and Ethical Issues in Medicine and Psychiatry*. New York: Oxford University Press.

Engelhardt, H. Tristram Jr. 1975. "The Concepts of Health and Disease." In *Evaluation and Explanation in the Biomedical Sciences*, edited by H. Tristram Engelhardt Jr. and Stuart F. Spicker (1st edn), 125–141. Dordrecht: D. Reidel Publishing Company.

Epicurus. 1966. "Letter to Menoeceus." In *Greek and Roman Philosophy after Aristotle*, edited by Jason L. Saunders. New York: Free Press.

Ereshefsky, Marc. 2009. "Defining 'Health' and 'Disease'." *Studies in History and Philosophy of Science* 40 (3): 221–227.

Federal Ministry of Justice and Consumer Protection. n.d. "German Criminal Code." Accessed April 3, 2023. http://www.gesetze-im-internet.de/index.html.

Fulford, William K. M. 1989. *Moral Theory and Medical Practice*. Cambridge: Cambridge University Press.

Gert, Bernard. 2005. *Morality: Its Nature and Justification*. Oxford: Oxford University Press.

Gert, Bernard, Charles M. Culver, and K. Danner Clouser. 2006. *Bioethics: A Systematic Approach* (2nd edn). Oxford: Oxford University Press.

Hucklenbroich, Peter. 2008. "'Normal - Anders - Krank': Begriffsklärungen und theoretische Grundlagen zum Krankheitsbegriff." In *Normal - Anders - Krank? Akzeptanz, Stigmatisierung und Pathologisierung im Kontext der Medizin*, edited by Dominik Groß, Sabine Müller, and Jan Steinmetzer, 3–31. Berlin: Medizinisch Wissenschaftliche Verlagsgesellschaft.

Jaster, Romy. 2020. *Agents' Abilities*. Berlin: De Gruyter.

Megone, Christopher. 2000. "Mental Illness, Human Function, and Values." *Philosophy, Psychiatry, and Psychology* 7 (1): 45–65.

Nordenfelt, Lennart. 1995. *On the Nature of Health an Action-Theoretic Approach* (2nd edn). Dordrecht: Springer.

———. 2001. *Health, Science, and Ordinary Language*. New York: Rodopi.

Reznek, Lawrie. 1987. *The Nature of Disease*. London: Routledge.

———. 1991. *The Philosophical Defence of Psychiatry*. Florence: Taylor and Francis/Routledge.

Schramme, Thomas. 2007. "A Qualified Defense of a Naturalist Theory of Health." *Medicine, Health Care and Philosophy* 10 (1): 11–17.

Thagard, Paul. 1999. *How Scientists Explain Disease*. Princeton: Princeton University Press.

Wakefield, Jerome C. 1992. "The Concept of Mental Disorder. On the Boundary between Biological Facts and Social Values." *American Psychologist* 47 (3): 373–388.

3 Biological Function Views

In Chapter 2, I have discussed the Harm Views and Action Views of the concept MENTAL DISORDER. In this chapter, I will reconstruct and evaluate two of the major prevalent Biological Function Views of the concept MENTAL DISORDER. These are the views of Wakefield (1992a, 1992b, 2006) and Boorse (1975, 1976a, 1977, 1997).[1] Roughly, the idea of these views is this: an individual has a mental disorder (if and) only if they are in a condition that results from a failure of some mental mechanism to perform at least one of its biological functions.[2] Wakefield's "Harmful Dysfunction Analysis" (HDA) and Boorse's "Biostatistical Theory" (BST) differ in the following respects:

1 their definition of "biological function" and, consequently, their view on what it is for a mechanism to "dysfunction" or to "fail" to perform its biological function (see Boorse 1976b, 2002; Wakefield 1992b, 1999) and
2 whether the presence of a biological dysfunction is not only necessary but also sufficient for having a mental disorder (in a theoretical sense of the term).

According to Wakefield (1992b, 2014), the presence of a biological dysfunction is not sufficient for an individual to have a mental disorder, but the presence of harm is necessary too. Boorse (1997) denies the latter claim when it comes to the presence of a mental disorder in a theoretical sense, but recognizes it for various practical senses of the term. Given that I am interested in explicating MENTAL DISORDER for theoretical *and* practical purposes, the main difference between HDA and BST lies in difference (1): Wakefield's and Boorse's definitions of "biological function." Boorse offers a goal-directed system definition of "biological function," whereas Wakefield offers an evolutionary one.

This chapter is structured as follows.[3] In Section 3.1, I elaborate on the concept MECHANISM because it plays an important role in Biological

DOI: 10.4324/9781003367840-4

Function Views. In Sections 3.2 and 3.3, I reconstruct Wakefield's HDA and Boorse's BST. I also discuss some problems with their views. In Section 3.4, I evaluate Biological Function Views in light of the adequacy conditions outlined in Section 1.3.

3.1 Mechanisms

The concept MECHANISM is primarily invoked in explanations (see Krickel 2018).[4] An explanation has an explanandum (a description of that which is to be explained) and an explanans (a description of that which explains). In a mechanistic explanation, we refer to a mechanism to explain a phenomenon that is to be explained. If we want to know what mechanisms are, we must examine how we use the term "mechanism" in the context of its explanatory role. This role involves explaining the phenomenon that is to be explained by describing (1) a phenomenon type, (2) a mechanism type, and (3) the relation that obtains between them.

According to mechanists (such as Machamer, Darden, and Craver 2000, Craver 2007, and Bechtel 2008), a MECHANISM is a system of causally interacting parts organized such that they are *responsible* for the phenomenon to be explained. This is called the "minimal characterization" of MECHANISM.[5] One implication of this characterization is that mechanisms are identified relative to the phenomenon for which they are responsible. According to Carl Craver (2007), what demarcates the entities that form components of a mechanism from those that do not is whether they are (either causally or constitutively) relevant to the phenomenon they are responsible for. Different types of mechanisms are individuated in virtue of the different types of phenomena for which they are responsible. For example, the BLOOD-PUMP-ING MECHANISM is defined as the mechanism responsible for pumping blood through an organism. The (hypothetical) FEAR MECHANISM is defined as the mechanism responsible for fear in an organism. In short, as Stuart Glennan (1996) puts it, a mechanism is always a mechanism *for* a phenomenon.

According to Wesley Salmon (1984), there are two kinds of mechanistic explanations. That is, there are two ways to understand what it means to be "responsible" for a phenomenon: etiological explanations and constitutive explanations. In an etiological explanation, the explanandum is explained by the mechanism (under a description) that consists of the *preceding causes* of the phenomenon. In a constitutive explanation, the explanandum is explained by the mechanism (under a description) that *underlies* or *constitutes* the phenomenon. *Prima facie*, a mechanistic explanation differs from a deductive-nomological explanation (see Hempel and Oppenheim 1948) because it does not rely on deduction and descriptions of laws. Rather, it relies on descriptions of either causal or constitutive relations between the phenomenon and the mechanism.

For the most part, etiological mechanisms and phenomena are taken to be sorts of events or causal sequences of events. This is because the relationship between an etiological mechanism and the phenomenon they are responsible for is a causal one, and, arguably, only events can stand in causal relations.[6] Roughly, etiological mechanisms are sequences of events that causally result in a phenomenon to be explained. Krickel (2018) argues that this characterization is trivial because it renders virtually all causal sequences of events as mechanisms. Nonetheless, for present purposes, we do not need to provide a full definition of ETIOLOGICAL MECHANISM. It suffices to know that etiological mechanisms are causal sequences of events that cause a phenomenon to be explained + X.

In light of this, there are at least two options for what is "mental" about a "mental mechanism." The *mechanism* itself or the *phenomenon* the mechanism is responsible for could be "mental." According to Boorse, mental health is "the special case obtained by focusing on the functions of *mental processes*" (1976a, 63, my emphasis). Arguably, both the mechanism and the phenomenon are processes. It is therefore unclear whether Boorse considers the mechanism or the phenomenon to be mental. According to Wakefield, it is not necessary that the mechanism itself be mental; "to be mental, the underlying dysfunction need only be a failure of the biologically designed function of some mechanism to *produce or regulate mental states*" (2006, 127, my emphasis). Hence, for Wakefield, a mental mechanism can either be a mechanism that is itself mental or a mechanism that is responsible for a mental phenomenon. I return to this issue in Section 3.4.

Mechanisms can "fail" or "break," that is, not produce the phenomenon they are responsible for. But, herein lies a problem. If a mechanism X is *defined* by the phenomenon X it causes, then a mechanism that *fails* to produce a phenomenon X is not a mechanism X at all. For instance, the (hypothetical) FEAR MECHANISM is defined as the mechanism that causes the phenomenon of fear. If a mechanism fails to cause fear, then it does not fall under FEAR MECHANISM. It is inconsistent to claim that a mechanism occurred but failed to produce the phenomenon it is responsible for. So, what is it to claim that a mechanism can "fail" or "break"? Krickel (2018, 55) argues that, strictly speaking, mechanism *tokens* cannot fail to cause the phenomenon they are responsible for. It is only mechanism *types* that can fail to be instantiated. On this view, to claim that a mechanism fails is to claim that a token of that mechanism did not occur in a circumstance in which it was, in some sense, "expected" to occur. Applied to fear, to claim that the fear mechanism "failed" is to claim that fear did not occur in a circumstance in which fear was, in some sense, "expected" to occur.

Some mechanisms can have biological functions. One prominent view (Cummins 1975; Millikan 1989; Neander 1991) holds that functions are taken to relate some entity to an effect. With the distinction between causal mechanisms and constitutive mechanisms in question, the biological function of a mechanism will be something that the mechanism either *causes* or *constitutes*.[7] Plausibly, when a mechanism has a biological function, then its biological function is identical to causing or constituting that phenomenon according to which the mechanism is defined. For instance, the BLOOD-PUMPING MECHANISM is defined as the mechanism that either causes or constitutes blood-pumping through an organism. If the circulation mechanism has a biological function, then it will be precisely to pump blood through an organism.

3.2 Wakefield

In this section, I will first reconstruct Wakefield's HDA and, second, discuss some problems specific to his view.

3.2.1 Reconstruction

Wakefield's HDA of MENTAL DISORDER was originally presented in two papers (1992a, 1992b). It can be reconstructed as follows:

HDA   An individual S has a mental disorder if and only if S is in a condition C that results from a failure of a mental mechanism to perform at least one of its proper biological functions and C is harmful by the standards of S's culture.

For illustration, consider anxiety disorder. According to HDA, an individual S has an anxiety disorder if and only if (1) S is in a condition that results from a failure of the fear mechanism to perform its proper biological function, and (2) this condition is harmful by the standards of S's culture. In Section 3.1, I stated that the FEAR MECHANISM is defined as the mechanism responsible for the phenomenon of fear. If a fear mechanism has a proper biological function, then that function is either to cause or to constitute fear. That a fear mechanism fails to perform its proper biological function is to say that fear does not occur in S in a circumstance in which it is, in some sense, expected to occur.

Let me now elaborate on "harm," "proper biological function," and the sense in which some phenomenon is "expected" to occur in Wakefield's HDA.

Wakefield offers several slightly different descriptions of the harm condition. A dysfunction counts as a disorder if and only if it causes "significant harm to the person under present environmental circumstances and according to present cultural standards" (Wakefield 1992a, 383–384). In addition, "*harmful* is a value term referring to the consequences that occur to the person because of the dysfunction and are deemed negative by socio-cultural standards" (Wakefield 1992a, 374). "[O]nly dysfunctions that are socially disvalued are disorders," and a condition is a disorder if and only if the condition "causes harm or deprivation of benefit to the person as judged by the standards of the person's culture" (Wakefield 1992a, 384).

However, as Neil Feit points out, it is unclear whether HDA makes use of "*social judgments about harm* instead of *harm itself* (so that, for example, a disorder need not be harmful, but simply disvalued by social norms)" (2017, 370). Charitably, Wakefield's view is this: S's condition C is harmful if and only if the standards of S's culture determine that C is harmful. So, if there was a culture wherein the relevant standards determine that epilepsy is not harmful, then epilepsy would not be harmful, and it would therefore not be a disorder. In this sense, harm, and consequently disorder, is culturally relative. On this interpretation of Wakefield's view, something is a harm relative to a culture whose standards determine that it is a harm.

Wakefield also considers ascriptions of functions to be teleological. To ascribe to X a function F is to state that X is in some sense "supposed" to F or that X was in some sense "designed" to F. Ruth Millikan (1989) and Karen Neander (1991) call "functions" (in this teleological sense) "proper functions." For Wakefield, it is only in virtue of having a proper function that an entity can dysfunction. In an organism, a "dysfunction exists only when an organ cannot perform as it is naturally (that is, independently of human intentions) supposed to perform" (Wakefield 1992a, 381).

It is well known that ascribing purposes to biological entities is problematic, whereas ascribing proper functions to artifacts is relatively unproblematic. This is because artifacts are typically made by individuals with certain intentions, whereas biological entities are not. In the case of artifacts, the proper function of an artifact corresponds to some of the intentions with which it was made. For instance, spectacles are made with the intention to make us see better. Presumably, the producer also had other intentions (for example, to make a profit). Which one of their intentions is the defining one? Plausibly, the function of spectacles is to make the wearer see better. But even if the answer is not clear, one of the producer's intentions will be the defining one. However, when it comes to biological entities, there are no intentions to begin with. So, to justify ascriptions of proper functions to biological entities (within a framework of the natural sciences), we need an explication of PROPER BIOLOGICAL FUNCTION in non-intentional terms.

Wakefield (1992a) specifies that "proper biological function" is to be understood in evolutionary terms, that is, in the sense of a naturally selected effect.[8] Neander offers the following explication of PROPER BIOLOGICAL FUNCTION (PBF):

PBF   It is the/a proper [biological] function of an item (X) of an organ-
       ism (O) to do that which items of X's type did to contribute to the
       inclusive fitness of O's ancestors, and which caused the genotype,
       of which X is the phenotypic expression, to be selected by natural
       selection.[9]

                                                                (1991, 174)

To clarify, a genotype is the set of genes an individual possesses. Genes can
be expressed as traits in an individual. A phenotype is the set of traits an
individual possesses. An individual's phenotype is determined not only by
their genes but also by environmental influences. Arguably, natural selection
operates on the phenotype (more specifically, on the variation of pheno-
types). It is the phenotype that gives an individual advantages or disadvantages in the struggle for survival and reproduction. And, a phenotype gives
only *relative* advantages or disadvantages (relative to other variations in a
population). A trait can be selected because of its effects only if having an
effect counts as an adaptive variation in the population. However, what
evolves is the genetic setup (see Dawkins 1976). Roughly put, evolution is
the change in a genotype as a result of the natural selection of a phenotype.

So, two of the basic assumptions of natural selection are that (1) variation in a trait is possible and (2) a given trait can be inherited (it can be
passed on to the next generation via the transmission of genes). Heritability is a measure of how much of the variance of a trait in a population is
accounted for by genetic variance. If the variation in the population is attributable to environmental influences alone, then any advantage will not
be passed on to the next generation. Traits that are passed on to the next
generation through nurture (for example, knowledge of historical events)
are not inherited but rather acquired traits.

In light of this, a trait can possess a PBF only if there were variations of
that trait in a population and the trait is transmitted genetically. Consequently, we should be cautious about ascribing PBFs to behavioral traits.
Unless behavioral traits can be explicitly linked to genes, any statement
regarding heritability, and therefore the trait's PBF, should be considered
suspect.

Applied to the FEAR MECHANISM, the following holds: if past mechanisms falling under FEAR MECHANISM were selected for either causing or
constituting the phenomenon of fear, then today's mechanisms falling under the FEAR MECHANISM have the PBF of either causing or constituting
fear. More precisely, a mechanism falling under FEAR MECHANISM has the
PBF to either cause or constitute fear only if fear contributed to the inclusive fitness of the organism's ancestors. This, in turn, caused the genotype
(of which fear is the phenotypic expression) to be selected by natural
selection.

Wakefield's HDA of MENTAL DISORDER can be reconstructed in more detail as follows:

HDA* An individual S has a mental disorder if and only if

> i   S has an organism that has a *mental mechanism* of type F as a component part;
>
> ii it is the *PBF* of the mental mechanism of type F to either cause or constitute F. That is,
>
>> tokens of F occurred in S's ancestors and caused the genotypes of which a token of F is the phenotypic expression to be naturally selected;
>
> iii S is in a condition C that results from, at least, one *dysfunction* of the mental mechanism of type F to perform F. That is,
>
>> a token of F does not occur in a circumstance in which it was "expected" to occur (and tokens of F used to occur in such circumstances in S's ancestors). Instead, some other event, process, or mechanism occurs that causes S's condition C; and
>
> iv C is *harmful* to S in the sense that the standards of S's culture determine that C is harmful.

Before evaluating HDA*, let me make a clarification on method. Should we conceive of HDA* as a conceptual analysis or an explication of the concept associated with the term "mental disorder"? Wakefield (2021, 284) admits that he has been somewhat "sloppy" about this question in some of his writings.[10] Recently, he has clarified that he thinks of HDA* as a two-step approach:

> "Harmful dysfunction" is a conceptual analysis prior to the evolutionary interpretation of "dysfunction," and the evolutionary interpretation of "function" is an essentialist theoretical move [...].
>
> (Wakefield 2021, 282)

So, on Wakefield's view, the first step is a conceptual analysis of "mental disorder," the outcome of which is that "disorder" means "harmful dysfunction." The second step is an explication of "function" and "dysfunction" in terms of evolutionary theory. The rationale for this explication is an inference to the best explanation: evolutionary theory provides us with the scientific theory that best explains the nature of functions and dysfunctions. In the end, HDA* is thus, at least in part, an explication of "mental disorder."

Wakefield has good reasons to conceive of HDA* as an explication. If we conceived of it as a conceptual analysis, then it would be extensionally inadequate. This is because—as has been argued in the literature and as I argue now—the presence of a biological dysfunction in terms of PBFs is not necessary for having a mental disorder.

3.2.2 *Evaluation*

There is a large amount of critical literature on HDA*, and Wakefield has offered comprehensive responses.[11] In this section, I focus on the arguments against (1) Wakefield's specific conception of HARM and (2) the necessity of "biological dysfunctions" in terms of PBFs for the presence of a mental disorder. These are the most relevant arguments to the project of explication I am pursuing. (I discuss the necessity of harm in Chapters 4 and 5. I argued against the sufficiency of harm in Chapter 2.)

Harm. Feit (2017) argues convincingly that Wakefield's cultural relativism about harm is problematic. I shall briefly discuss two of Feit's arguments.

First, different sub-cultures might have different values (Feit 2017, 370). Society at large might disvalue the conditions that pro-anorexia groups value. Whose values should be relevant in determining whether a condition falls under MENTAL DISORDER? Cultural relativism does not offer any help in settling such disagreements. To the contrary, it appears that we would have to accept that there is no general agreement on that question.

Second, Feit states that it "seems odd that one can be harmed [...] merely because others think she is harmed" (2017, 371).[12] This may be an understatement. It seems highly implausible that "X is harmful" is determined merely by the fact that people "believe X to be harmful." Or, in Susan Wolf's words, "[i]f an individual's valuing something isn't sufficient to give the thing real value [...] it is hard to see why a group's endorsement should carry any more weight" (2010, 46). There is an important sense in which drugs, alcohol, and cigarettes are harmful to their consumers regardless of whether anyone believes them to be harmful. Smoking kills even if you live in a society that idealizes smoking. Furthermore, as Feit (2017, 371) points out, one can be harmed without knowing it (and, I would add, mistaken about it). To be fair, Wakefield later concedes that "my ([1992a, 1992b]) claim that harm is judged by social values was overly simplistic" (2013, 1). He now suggests that the harm condition reflects "broader normative commitments, not just immediate social reactions" (Wakefield 2013, 2).

Biological Dysfunctions. Several authors argue that the presence of a "biological dysfunction" in terms of PBFs is not necessary for having a disorder (see Lilienfeld and Marino 1995, Murphy and Woolfolk 2000, Nordenfelt 2003, Cooper 2007, and Schwartz 2007). In the literature, the following five types of counterexamples are often discussed:

1 *Environmental Mismatches*: Disorders can be caused by mechanisms functioning in accordance with their PBF in circumstances in which that function is no longer adaptive.
2 *Inappropriate Input*: Disorders can be caused by mechanisms that are processing pathogenic input but doing so in accordance with their PBF.
3 *Exaptations*: Disorders can be caused by mechanisms that have shifted their PBF, that is, had some particular function in the past, but now have a different one.
4 *Spandrels*: Disorders can be caused by mechanisms that never had a PBF but are rather by-products of other mechanisms with such functions.
5 *Adaptations*: Disorders can be caused by mechanisms that are themselves adaptations.

In the following, I will discuss these putative counterexamples in turn. I argue that only (c), (d), and (e) are good counterexamples to Wakefield's view. Discussion of the other candidates is, though, instructive for explicating MENTAL DISORDER.

1 *Environmental Mismatches*[13]

Dominic Murphy and Robert Woolfolk (2000, 244) argue that, in some disorders, a mental or bodily mechanism may simply no longer be adaptive in its bearers' current environment. Their examples are light skin or high levels of aggressiveness in males (2000, 244). Murphy and Woolfolk argue that, in the current environment, these traits are just like smoke detectors placed too close to a stove. There is nothing intrinsically defective with such a smoke detector, it is just that it is unfavorably positioned. Similarly, there need not be a dysfunction in individuals with light skin or high levels of aggressiveness; they are just in an "unfavorable" environment.

However, neither light skin nor a high level of aggressiveness *per se* are considered disorders. According to Wakefield (2000, 257), this is precisely because there is nothing intrinsically defective with individuals possessing these traits. Individuals with light skin or a high level of aggressiveness may, though, have a *disposition* or a statistically higher risk for particular disorders (for example, skin cancer or conduct disorder). Having a disposition for a disorder and having an actual disorder are not the same. If anything, high levels of aggressiveness and light skin are maladaptive traits or disadvantageous dispositions. More generally, that some previously adaptive trait or mechanism is not adaptive in the current environment is not sufficient for having a disorder. The desire for sweet and/or high-fat foods is adaptive in an environment in which there is food scarcity, but it is not adaptive in an environment in which such foods are easily accessible (Wakefield 2021, 544). In any case, the desire for sweet and high-fat foods is not a disorder in an environment in which there is no food scarcity.

This example shows that it is important to keep functions, adaptations, and adaptive traits (or mechanisms) separate. A trait is *adaptive* if it contributes to the fitness of the organism that possesses it in the organism's *current* environment (relative to other types of traits in the population). It is an *adaptation* if it has evolved owing to past contributions to fitness. Most traits are both, that is, they are adaptive adaptations. By definition, every adaptation was once an adaptive trait, but not all adaptations are still adaptive and not every adaptive trait is yet an adaptation. Functions, in Wakefield's sense, are necessarily adaptations of an organism to an environment, but they are not necessarily adaptive in the current environment. Thus, we should avoid speaking of "maladaptation." There are only adaptations or functions that are maladaptive in current contexts.

This is not to say that there cannot be mental disorders that represent environmental (or even developmental) mismatches. Rather, it is to say that representing such a mismatch is not sufficient for having a mental disorder. Justin Garson (2021, 504), for instance, argues that it is plausible to assume that some cases of generalized anxiety disorder (GAD) represent developmental mismatches. In other words, having a GAD was adaptive for some of their bearers in their (stressful) environment as a child, but is not adaptive for them anymore in their (non-stressful) environment as an adult. This is because GAD comes with an enhanced alertness to potential dangers (Garson 2021, 505), and it is better to be "safe than sorry" in certain environments. Nevertheless, although on point, this example does not show that some mental disorders represent mismatches *but not dysfunctions*.

2 Inappropriate Input
Murphy and Woolfolk (2000, 281) argue that disorders can be caused by mechanisms processing pathogenic input according to their PBFs. Disorders could be learned responses to pathogenic environments. For instance, a depressive disorder could be caused by a perfectionist attitude or a negative self-image. A trauma- or stress-related disorder could be a case of PBF "producing pathology in the face of unmanageable trauma" (Murphy and Woolfolk 2000, 281).

However, Wakefield (2000) argues that Murphy and Woolfolk have falsely assumed that, to have a dysfunction, some mechanism must be "broken." Wakefield (2000, 262) suggests that a dysfunction can be caused by a broken mechanism *or* by a false input (an input that the mechanism was not designed to respond to). Murphy and Woolfolk (2000), in turn, respond that a "failure to perform a function" and "dysfunction" are not the same. If they were, "then your legs would be dysfunctional if they were tied together so that you couldn't walk" (Murphy and Woolfolk 2000, 281).

This debate may benefit from the discussion of mechanisms from Section 3.1. Recall that a mechanism can only "fail" in the sense that a token mechanism does not occur in a circumstance in which it was, in some sense, "expected" to occur. Consider the following analogy. A vending machine is made for certain types of inputs only, say, €0.50, €1, or €2. What happens if we insert a false input? The consequences depend on the type of false input we insert. If we insert €0.20, then the vending mechanism will not occur. Most likely, the coin will just pass through the machine. However, in this case, it would not make sense to claim that the vending mechanism *failed* to occur given that it was not expected to occur (after all, it was not designed for €0.20). If we insert CHF 2 (Swiss franc), then the vending mechanism might occur (because CHF 2 is sufficiently similar in shape to €2) even though it was not designed for this type of input. If the vending mechanism occurred, then we would not conclude that the mechanism failed. Rather, we would conclude that we have learned something new about the mechanism, that it is not as fine-grained as we believed it to be. If we insert or jam in CHF 5, then the vending mechanism will also not occur. Again, it would not make sense to claim that the vending mechanism *failed* to occur given that it was not expected to occur. However, jamming in CHF 5 has different consequences than inserting €0.20. After inserting €0.20, subsequent normal inputs can still be processed without any problems. But, after inserting CHF 5, subsequent normal inputs can no longer be processed because CHF 5 will block the mechanism. We would presumably conclude that the mechanism is blocked or temporarily "broken," and that the vending mechanism is failing to perform its proper function. So, it seems that false input is "pathogenic" only in cases in which it causes the "breaking" or "blocking" of a mechanism.

What this analogy is supposed to show is that there is no difference between "failure of a mechanism to perform its proper function" and a "dysfunction." Both are cases in which a mechanism token does not occur in a circumstance in which it was expected to occur. However, there is a difference between a failure of a mechanism to perform its proper function and mere non-occurrence. If a mechanism was not expected to occur, then it merely did not occur. The difference between *failure* and *success* makes sense only if there is some standard (success conditions) against which the actual workings of a mechanism can be compared.

Let us return to cases of mental disorder. Can there be instances of mental disorder that result from a mechanism processing false inputs according to its PBF without there being a "broken" mechanism? One of Murphy and Woolfolk's (2000) examples is post-traumatic stress disorder (PTSD) in which proper biological functioning produces pathology in the face of unmanageable trauma. However, PTSD seems to be much closer to the CHF 5 case than to the €0.20 case in the vending machine analogy. If individuals did not have intense flashbacks after having experienced traumatic events, then they would not be considered as having PTSD. In these cases, we would think that the trauma *was manageable* after all. The fact that individuals with PTSD have intense flashbacks provides evidence that the mechanism is impaired when it comes to processing input for which it was "designed" according to its PBF.

In light of this, examples such as "legs being dysfunctional if they were tied together so that one couldn't walk" are not instances in which a mechanism *fails* to perform its function. The circumstances are not such that the mechanism is expected to occur. This example is better captured in terms of *abilities*, where some enabling condition to exercise the relevant ability is not met. If your legs are tied, then you do not lack your general ability to walk. You cannot walk because the situational conditions for exercising your general ability are not met. We might say that one's general ability to walk is "masked" by temporary obstacles.

3 Exaptations

Scott Lilienfeld and Lori Marino (1995) argue that there may be disorders of mental mechanisms that are exaptations. Exaptations are traits or mechanisms that were selected for one effect but shifted their function during the course of evolution (see Gould and Vrba 1982). The paradigmatic example is the feathering of birds, which is believed to originally have been selected for thermoregulation and later co-opted for flight. According to Lilienfeld and Marino (1995), there could be disorders that are caused by mechanisms that shifted their function. Such disorders had one PBF in the past but have a different one today.

Murphy and Woolfolk (2000) point out that Wakefield could accommodate exaptations by restricting his thesis to the latest evolutionary developments of the mind's architecture. What counts is not the mind's original PBF, but rather the most recent adaptations. However, this option comes with further difficulties. To have a PBF in Wakefield's sense, it is necessary that the trait or mechanism has a selective history. It must have been selected for its fitness-enhancing effect. Thus, new mutations with beneficial effects do not have PBFs (yet). It is possible nonetheless that there are disorders of such mechanisms.

Moreover, any conception of MENTAL DISORDER that relies on PBFs faces the following problem: where do the most recent PBFs end and currently beneficial effects begin? Any comprehensive conception of MENTAL DISORDER in terms of PBFs must somehow deal with this problem.

4 *Spandrels*

Stephen Gould and Richard Lewontin (1979) argue for the existence of so-called "spandrels." Spandrels are adventitious side effects of the development of certain functions that themselves never possessed any adaptive function. Gould and Lewontin (1979) hold that some traits may be such side effects. Given that "trait" might refer to any type of property of an organism (for example, snoring, the grumbling of the stomach, or the pounding of the heart), this claim is trivially true. The more interesting claim is that there might be spandrels (and even failures thereof) that cause pathological conditions. If there are spandrels of the mind (and failures thereof) that either cause or constitute mental disorders but are not also failures of a PBF, then not all mental disorders are dysfunctions in the evolutionary sense.

Wakefield's (2000, 254) reply is that nobody ever gave an *actual* example of a spandrel-inspired mental disorder. On his view, merely pointing out the possibility of such a case does not prove anything; it only asserts what must be shown. However, if we conceive of HDA* as a conceptual analysis of "mental disorder," then Wakefield's reply is problematic. Pointing out a hypothetical class of counterexamples is sufficient to show that the presence of a biological dysfunction is not *necessary* for having a mental disorder. It suffices to show that it is *conceivable* that there be a mental disorder without a biological dysfunction.

5 *Adaptations*

Murphy and Woolfolk (2000, 244) claim that some mental disorders such as depressive disorder may be adaptive mechanisms. Depression might be a fitness-enhancing way to conserve energy and to elicit aid from others and it might have been selected because of that, and thus have a biological function. So, on Murphy and Woolfolk's view, not all mental disorders necessarily involve biological dysfunctions.

Wakefield's (2000) reply is that intuitions about mental disorders such as depressive disorder depend on the intensity of the condition and that this, in turn, correlates with our intuitions about whether they are adaptive and have a biological function. On Wakefield's view, only moderate depressiveness could have been adaptive, and we do not generally consider moderate cases to be dysfunctions or disorders. Biological dysfunctions are attributed only to *extreme* cases in which they do "not appear to be useful strategies by any stretch of the imagination"

(Wakefield 2000, 260). So, for Wakefield, only some range on the continuum of depressiveness might have been selected for its beneficial effects, and what falls under DEPRESSIVE DISORDER is clearly out of this range.

But, again, if we conceive of HDA* as a conceptual analysis, then Wakefield's reply is problematic. Whether a certain genetic variant is selected for or against depends not only on the phenotype but also on which other variants exist in the population.[14] To clarify this point, imagine a population wherein individuals have either very high levels of fear or no fear at all. The chances of survival and reproduction may be low for individuals with high levels of fear, but those chances might still be higher than the chances of survival and reproduction for individuals with no fear at all. This is because, in evolutionary terms, it is better to be "safe than sorry." It is clearly more adaptive to be able to experience fear (for avoiding dangerous situations) than it is to lack this ability completely. Hence, it may be the case that extreme cases of fear (or depressiveness) were selected for their effects and possess a PBF after all. In any case, extreme fear (or depressiveness) is generally considered to be pathological.

Now, what if we conceive of HDA* as an explication? Because I am interested in an explication of MENTAL DISORDER for scientific and normative purposes, this seems to be the more pressing question. If we conceive of HDA* as an explication, then Wakefield can be revisionary about the conceivable counterexamples, and he can argue that we *should not* think of exaptations, spandrels, and adaptations as disorders. But, then, why should we (as theorists) restrict the concept of MENTAL DISORDER to biological dysfunctions defined in terms of PBFs in the first place? In the end, the biological dysfunction condition of HDA* is not a conceptual condition, but rather an empirical one. And, as we have seen when explicating PBFs, this condition is a highly demanding one given that it requires heritability. However, the relevance of the evolutionary perspective for the concept of MENTAL DISORDER is not evident.[15] Murphy (2020) points out that medicine does not make such a restriction. Jonathan Tsou (2021, 44) argues that it would be "pragmatically indefensible" for us (as members of society) to stop classifying depression or PTSD as mental disorders if it turned out that they were neither caused nor constituted by biological dysfunctions.

Now, Wakefield could argue that medicine should make such a restriction and that we should stop considering depression or PTSD as mental disorders if it turns out that they are neither caused nor constituted by biological dysfunctions defined in terms of PBFs. This is because this is what our best scientific theory of the nature of functions and dysfunctions yields, and our concept of MENTAL DISORDER depends on the concept of DYSFUNCTION. However, as I shall argue in Chapters 4 and 5, when it comes to mental disorder, there is an alternative view.

In any case, it is worth noting that HDA* has the following two drawbacks:

1   In light of HDA*, the status of the phenomena that scientists consider to be mental disorders is *preliminary* in the sense that the classification depends on our knowledge of the evolution of the mind; knowledge that is currently quite limited.
2   HDA* *restricts* the causal explanations of mental disorders because it depends on a highly demanding concept of biological dysfunction.

As long as scientists do not know enough about the evolution of the mind and the exact causes of mental disorders, a definition should remain neutral with respect to these issues. Moreover, defining MENTAL DISORDER is a conceptual project that "picks out" certain phenomena as a set. Finding out about the causes of mental disorders (that is, of the phenomena "picked out" by MENTAL DISORDER) is an empirical project that explains the occurrences of those phenomena. It is not the job of a definition to tell us about the causes of mental disorders and the evolution of the mind, but rather the job of the empirical sciences. A definition of MENTAL DISORDER that remains neutral (that is, is not committed to any particular explanation) on the evolution of the mind and the causes of mental disorders would be preferable. It would enable us to keep the projects of definition and explanation apart and remain open with respect to new empirical findings.

Let me make a last point here. Why is an analysis of the MENTAL DISORDER concept in terms of PBFs inadequate? Here is one explanation: Wakefield aims to analyze MENTAL DISORDER by means of a concept that was fashioned for a wholly different purpose. Recall the distinction between conceptual analysis and explication, the former being a descriptive and the latter a revisionary project (see Section 1.1). The concept PBF is not the result of a conceptual analysis. Millikan writes as follows:

> Proper function is intended as a technical term. It is of interest because it can be used to unravel certain problems, not because it does or doesn't accord with common notions such as "purpose" or the ordinary notion "function." My program is far removed from conceptual analysis; I need a term that will do a certain job and so I must fashion one.
>
> (1984, 2)

It appears that the concept PBF was designed to solve certain problems in evolutionary biology and not in psychiatry or clinical psychology. This should give us reason to be wary of using the concept PBF in an explication of MENTAL DISORDER.

3.3 Boorse

In this section, I will first reconstruct Boorse's BST and, second, discuss some problems specific to his view.

3.3.1 Reconstruction

Boorse formulates his BST of HEALTH and DISEASE (in my terminology: DISORDER) as follows:

BST
1. The *reference class* is a natural class of organisms of uniform functional design; specifically, i.e., an age group of a sex of a species.
2. A *normal [physiological] function* of an internal part or process within members of a reference class is its statistically typical contribution to survival or reproduction.[16]
3. *Health* in a member of a reference class is normal functional ability: the readiness of each internal part to perform its normal functions on typical occasions with typical efficiency.[17]
4. A *disease* or *pathological condition* is an internal state which impairs health, i.e., reduces one or more functional abilities below typical efficiency.

(Boorse 2014, 684)[18]

According to Boorse, BST is an analysis of both BODILY DISORDER and MENTAL DISORDER. He proposes the following view:

A mental disturbance gets classed as "mental illness" when some accepted explanation of it refers not to the patient's physiology but to his feelings, beliefs, and experiences. The defining property of mental disease is mental causation.

(Boorse 1976a, 67)

For the purposes of this chapter, we can assume that on Boorse's view the mental health-relevant mechanisms are mental ones (regardless of how exactly those are to be understood). Nothing in my critical evaluation of BST hinges on a specific account of what makes a mechanism a "mental" one.

For illustration, let us consider anxiety disorder again. According to BST, an individual S has an anxiety disorder if and only if S is in a condition C wherein the efficiency of the normal physiological function of S's fear mechanism is reduced below typical efficiency (compared with the relevant reference class). As before, the FEAR MECHANISM is defined as the mechanism responsible for the phenomenon of fear. If a fear mechanism has a normal physiological function, then it is, roughly, to either cause or constitute fear.

Let me now elaborate on "normal physiological function," "typical efficiency," and the basic framework of Boorse's BST.

According to Boorse (1977), the bearers of disorders are organisms. For something to be an organism, it is necessary that it has parts that are organized in a particular way. It is the physiological organization of an organism that matters for ascriptions of health and disorder. The physiology of any organism is a hierarchy of goal-directed systems.

Boorse is well aware that "goal-directedness" has a mental reading, something like "what I aim for." On this reading, a system can only be goal-directed if it has mental states like desires and intentions. However, not all organisms have mental states (for example, plants), and neither do sub-systems of organisms (for example, the brain or cardiovascular system). To solve this problem, Boorse (1977, 555) suggests that we adopt the conception of GOAL-DIRECTED SYSTEM endorsed by Gerd Sommerhoff (1950, 1959) and Ernest Nagel (1961). Thus,

[a] physical system has the purely physical, nonintensional, property of being directed to a goal G when disposed to adjust its behavior, through some range of environmental variation, in ways needed to achieve G.

(Boorse 2011, 27)

Boorse seems to believe that for an organism to be directed toward some goal simply is to have some type of disposition, period.[19] (However, his own description reveals that what he refers to is not a mere disposition, but a disposition *to achieve a goal G*. Hence, although Boorse would like to get rid of the teleology problem, he does not succeed in doing so.)[20]

Arguably, organisms can have many "goals" or dispositions concurrently (for example, individual survival, individual reproduction, species survival, gene survival, and ecological equilibrium). Boorse (1977, 556) contends that in physiology, the relevant highest-level goals of the organism as a whole are individual survival and reproduction. Thus, because health is concerned with physiology, and physiology is concerned with individual survival and reproduction, health is concerned with individual survival and reproduction.

According to Boorse, a function is simply "a contribution to a goal" of a goal-directed system (1976b, 70).[21] More specifically, functions are causal contributions, and their bearers are the parts, processes, or mechanisms of a goal-directed system (Boorse 1976b, 77 f.). Every goal of a goal-directed system can serve to generate statements about functions (1976b, 77).[22] On Boorse's view, physiological function statements and physiology in general are not primarily concerned with individual organisms, but rather with a class of them:

the physiological functions of a part-type are its typical causal contributions to individual survival and reproduction in a whole species, or fraction thereof in the case of function limited to one age (bone growth) or sex (lactation).

(2011, 27)

Boorse's conception of a NORMAL PHYSIOLOGICAL FUNCTION (NPF) can be reconstructed as follows:

NPF   A mechanism of an organism has a *normal physiological function* F if and only if

  i   it is normal for the members of the class of organisms O to have a mechanism that either causes or constitutes F and
  ii F contributes causally to the individual survival or reproduction of the members of O.

The cardiovascular system, for instance, has the NPF to pump blood through an organism on statistically normal occasions with at least statistically normal efficiency. This is because (i) doing so contributes to the individual survival and/or reproduction of the organism, and (ii) it is, statistically speaking, what cardiovascular systems normally do.

Notice that statistics play a triple role in BST:

1 only those mechanisms are relevant that the members of the reference class statistically normally *possess*;
2 the relevant mechanisms occur on *occasions* that are statistically normal (or not); and
3 the relevant mechanisms occur with an *efficiency* that is statistically normal (or not).

Now, it is important to keep apart (a) the *process* of pumping blood through an organism and (b) the *NPF* of the cardiovascular system to pump blood through the organism (on normal occasions and with, at least, normal efficiency). Of course, an individual can have a disorder if their cardiovascular system pumps too much blood through them (and not only if it pumps too little). But, if we are talking about efficiency, then an individual whose cardiovascular system is more efficient at pumping blood does not have a disorder. Because NPF is defined in terms of efficiency, an individual is healthy only if their mechanisms perform their NPFs with "at least statistically typical efficiency, i.e. at efficiency levels *within or above* some chosen central region of their population distribution" (Boorse 1977, 558 f., my emphasis).

Boorse's BST of MENTAL DISORDER can be reconstructed in more detail as follows:

BST*   An individual S has a mental disorder if and only if

    i   S has an organism (being a member of a certain reference class within a class of organisms R) that has a *mental mechanism* of type F as a component part;

    ii   it is the *NPF* of the mental mechanism of type F to either cause or constitute F. That is,

        a   it is statistically normal for members of R to have a mental mechanism that either causes or constitutes F;

        b   F contributes causally to the individual survival or reproduction of the members of R; and

    iii a token of F does not occur on normal occasions C with, at least, the *efficiency* that is statistically normal for the members of R.

3.3.2 Evaluation

As with the HDA*, there is a large amount of critical literature on BST*, much of which Boorse has responded to.[23] In this section, I will focus on two arguments against the claim that the presence of a biological dysfunction is necessary and sufficient for the presence of a mental disorder.

1   *Not Necessary*. One problem for BST is that it does not capture *universal* (and common) *disorders* (Neander 1991, Melander 1997, Schwartz 2007, Kraemer 2013). In fact, BST implies that a universal biological dysfunction is conceptually impossible. But this is false. Conceptually, it is possible that all tokens of a certain type of entity have a biological function while not functioning properly. An understanding of the concept associated with the term "biological function" that does not capture this conceptual intuition will be inadequate. Peter Melander offers the following example:

> If reticulum cancer were to become pandemic in the bovine population thereby making all or most bovine reticulums unable to break down cellulose, bovine reticulums would not typically or normally be able to break down cellulose. But contrary to the proposal, to break down cellulose would then still be a function of bovine reticulums.
>
> (1997, 57)

Neander argues along similar lines that BST yields an absurd consequence: "if enough of us are stricken with disease (roughly, are dysfunctional) we cease to be diseased, which is nonsense" (1991, 182).

Even if we all go blind, blindness will still be a dysfunction. On Neander's view, it is conceptually possible that a biological dysfunction affects all members of a class of organisms. Spreading a disease does not make the condition any less of a disease.

Paul Griffiths and John Matthewson (2018) argue likewise that Boorse cannot account for diseases of old age (for example, ostheoarthritis). Given that the relevant reference class is an age group of a sex in a species, they argue, "deleterious physical states that become widespread at certain ages will not be classed as dysfunctional" (2018, 313).

Boorse (2002, 95) replies that vital biological dysfunctions, if universal, would simply extinguish the species. Even if this is true, it is not impossible for an entire species to fall ill with a deadly disorder. Nonetheless, Boorse thinks that only less-than-vital universal disorders are a threat to his view because there are *de facto* no vital universal disorders. For capturing less-than-vital universal disorders, Boorse claims that we must "use an extended time-slice of the species" (2002, 95) to determine those mechanisms that are normal for members of a species to have. The NPFs of a species are determined not only by the currently living members of that species but also by a set of past members. So, for some mechanism to have an NPF, it must have had the trait for a sufficient period of time. How long is sufficient though? According to Boorse,

> any time-slice shorter than a lifetime or two seems too short for the very idea of a species-typical functional design, since identifying many functions in maturation and reproduction requires a longitudinal view of an individual organism and its progeny.
>
> (2002, 99)

Boorse recognizes that this is somewhat vague, but thinks that vagueness is inevitable at some point.

Interestingly, Boorse's proposal for less-than-vital universal disorders indicates that our ascriptions of biological functions do not ultimately track statistical normality, but rather traits that have been beneficial to our ancestors. Identifying NPFs with respect to time-slices of a certain species may be a way to identify some of the PBFs that contributed to the inclusive fitness of a species. This makes sense given that one would expect that a trait in a class of organisms is statistically normal because it has a biological function and not the other way around.

There is another reason for believing that the presence of a biological dysfunction in terms of NPFs is not necessary for having a mental disorder. Tsou points out that certain mental disorders "might turn out to be underwritten by biological mechanisms that behave in predictable ways, but fall within the (statistically) normal range of biological functioning" (2021, 31).[24] This echoes the spandrel objection raised against the HDA* (see Section 3.2). It seems that we simply do not know enough about the causes of mental disorders to evaluate whether the phenomena falling under our actual MENTAL DISORDER concept are caused by biological dysfunctions in terms of NPFs. In light of this, a definition of MENTAL DISORDER that remains neutral with respect to the causes of mental disorders seems preferable.

2   *Not Sufficient.* Critics such as Rachel Cooper (2005, 17) and Andreas Heinz (2014, 44) argue that BST must be refuted because it falsely implies that homosexuality is a mental disorder. But this is only approximately true. BST might imply that homosexuality is a mental disorder if the following were true: in homosexual individuals, the mental mechanism responsible for heterosexual desire is not instantiated on statistically normal occasions with, at least, the efficiency that is statistically normal for the members of the relevant reference class. However, the argument would go, either causing or constituting heterosexual desire is the NPF of that mechanism. This is because it is statistically normal for members of the relevant reference class to have that mechanism, and having heterosexual desires contributes causally to the individual survival or reproduction of the members of the relevant reference class.

The crucial (empirical) question is whether there actually is a mental mechanism responsible for heterosexual desire. If there were, then BST would imply that homosexuality is a mental disorder. Boorse does not consider this problematic because (1) empirically, the question is not settled and (2) even if empirical research indicated that there is such a mechanism, this would indicate only that homosexuality falls under a *theoretical* concept associated with the term "disorder." But, because statistical normality does not entail desirability, this would have no practical significance. In sum, Boorse's view is that categorizing homosexuality as a mental disorder is unproblematic because it does not imply that homosexuality is undesirable. According to the BST, having a mental disorder is about functional statistical normality and not at all about desirability.

What should we make of this? Boorse is interested in an analysis of the theoretical concept associated with the term "disorder." But homosexuality is not considered a mental disorder in clinical psychology or psychiatry. BST is thus inadequate as an analysis of our actual theoretical concept associated with the term "mental disorder." Our view is not that scientists do not have sufficient empirical evidence to know whether homosexuality is a mental disorder. Rather, it is that homosexuality is not a mental disorder, not even in a theoretical sense of the term.

If one is interested in an explication of MENTAL DISORDER, as I am in this book, this leaves open the question of whether we *should* consider homosexuality a mental disorder. Here, the answer is "no."[25] Being homosexual does not give the individual a *pro tanto* reason to seek psychiatric or psychotherapeutic treatment (if available). The fact that someone is homosexual is not worthy of psychiatric or psychotherapeutic concern (although the fact that they are subject to stigmatization might be).

Another example showing that the presence of a biological dysfunction in terms of NPFs is not sufficient for having a mental disorder is *diminished jealousy*. According to BST, an individual would have a mental disorder if there was a mechanism for jealousy instantiated in them on statistically normal occasions with less than statistically normal intensity. However, diminished jealousy is not a mental disorder and should not be considered one because it is not worthy of psychiatric or psychotherapeutic concern.

3.4 Biological Function Views Evaluated

In this section, I will evaluate Wakefield's HDA* and Boorse's BST* in light of the adequacy conditions outlined in Section 1.3.

As a preliminary, note the following about the relationship between PBF and NPF. PBFs relate to the "goals" of the units of evolution, whereas NPFs relate to the "goals" of individual organisms in a species. Chances are high, however, that these concepts' extensions overlap. We can expect that PBFs will become statistically normal in a (reference class of a) species, and that many of them contribute to the survival and reproduction of individual organisms. Furthermore, the relevant timespan for ascribing the respective functions will be similar. In HDA*, we are interested in PBFs given the most recent evolutionary developments of the mind's architecture. In BST*, we are interested in NPFs given an extended time-slice of a species. Because statistics follow function and not the other way around, it is reasonable to assume that some NPFs track a subset of PBFs. However, not all NPFs will track PBFs because the former need not be hereditary in the sense required for ascriptions of the latter.

3.4.1 *Mental Disorder versus Mental Health*

The evaluations in Sections 3.2 and 3.3 suggest that Biological Function Views are extensionally inadequate with respect to some clear cases of mental health and mental disorders. As such, Biological Function Views do not adequately explicate MENTAL DISORDER. More specifically, the presence of a biological dysfunction—either in terms of PBFs or NPFs—is neither necessary nor sufficient for having a mental disorder.

The presence of a biological dysfunction in terms of PBFs is not necessary for having a mental disorder because it is conceptually possible that there are disorders of exaptations or spandrels. It is also conceptually possible that disorders can be adaptations. The presence of a biological dysfunction in terms of NPFs is not necessary for having a mental disorder because it is conceptually possible that there be disorders of mechanisms that behave in predictable ways but fall within the statistically normal range of biological functioning. The presence of a biological dysfunction in terms of NPFs is also not sufficient for having a mental disorder because such a view could falsely imply that homosexuality or diminished jealousy are mental disorders.

More generally, we should not explicate MENTAL DISORDER in terms of biological dysfunctions because the projects of *definition* and *explanation* need to be kept separate. They also need to remain open with respect to new empirical findings about the (biological) structure of the mind. That said, an explication of MENTAL DISORDER should be open to the possibility that at least some cases of MENTAL DISORDER are either caused or constituted by biological dysfunctions. Certain types of explanations should not be excluded by definition.

3.4.2 Mental Disorder versus Bodily Disorder

According to HDA* and BST*, the distinction between MENTAL DISORDER and BODILY DISORDER is analyzed by the type of mechanism that is failing to perform its PBF or NPF, respectively. Mental disorders involve mental mechanisms, while bodily disorders involve bodily mechanisms that fail to perform their biological functions. Furthermore, in case all types of mental mechanisms have corresponding types of bodily mechanisms, we could argue that there is ultimately no interesting difference between mental mechanisms and bodily mechanisms. This is a *prima facie* plausible view.

But BODILY MECHANISM and MENTAL MECHANISM need to be analyzed further. Recall that there are, at least, two ways in which a mental mechanism could be mental. A mechanism could be mental in virtue of (a) the fact that the *phenomenon* it causes or constitutes is mental or (b) the fact that the *mechanism* itself is mental. When we evaluate whether a certain type of disorder is mental or bodily, we might get different results depending on which of these views we adopt.

Consider somatic symptom disorder. The diagnostic criteria for somatic symptom disorder include both (1) the presence of somatic symptoms (without the presence of a bodily disorder) and (2) the individual's worrying about their somatic symptoms, which is a mental phenomenon. Now, imagine a case in which an individual has somatic symptoms without either the presence of a bodily disorder or any worry about their somatic symptoms. Does the affected individual have a mental disorder (if they have a disorder at all)? A Biological Function View yields different results depending on which view of mental mechanisms we adopt. If a mental mechanism is a mechanism that either causes or constitutes a mental phenomenon, then a Biological Function View implies that the phenomenon is not a *mental* disorder (if it is a disorder at all). This is because the relevant phenomenon—having bodily symptoms—is not a mental one. If a mental mechanism is a mental mechanism that either causes or constitutes some phenomenon, then a Biological Function View implies that the phenomenon is a mental disorder (if it is a disorder at all).

Moreover, there are various views on what properties constitute the "mental" (for example, intentionality and/or phenomenal consciousness). Any analysis of MENTAL MECHANISM will have to elaborate on this issue.

3.4.3 Mental Disorder versus Deviance from Social, Legal, or Moral Norms

Can a Biological Function View account for the difference between mental disorders and deviance from social, legal, or moral norms? It seems that it can because it refers to a "biological norm" that differs from social, legal, or moral norms in relevant ways. According to HDA*, the biological norm is given by the evolutionary history of a mechanism: it is that which contributed to the inclusive fitness of the organism's ancestors. According to BST*, the biological norm is the statistically normal contribution of a certain set of mechanisms to the goals of an organism that are of interest to us in the medical context (namely, individual survival and reproduction).

In light of this, the relationship between having a mental disorder and deviating from a social, legal, or moral norm, can be captured as follows:

a   cases of *mere social, legal, or moral deviance* are such that one only violates a social, legal, or moral norm, but does not depart from a "biological norm";

b   cases of *mere mental disorder* are such that one only departs from a "biological norm," but does not violate a social, legal, or moral norm;

c   cases of *mental disorder and social, legal, or moral deviance* are such that one departs from a "biological norm" *and* violates a social, legal, or moral norm.

Two clarifications are necessary.

First, the concept NPF is, in some sense, dependent on society because interests play a role in its determination. This does not imply decisionism about NPFs, however. In a medical context, once the goals that interest us are fixed, what falls under the concept NORMAL PHYSIOLOGICAL DYSFUNC-TION will be determined independently of our choices.

Second, biological norms differ from social, legal, or moral norms in that they are not prescriptive. The "norm" in "biological norm" is a teleological standard. That some mechanism deviates from a biological norm—that is, from a certain "goal"—does not, by itself, give us any reason to do something about it.

3.4.4 Normative Purposes

That a mechanism is not performing its PBF or NPF does not, by itself, entail any normative consequences. As stated earlier, biological norms are not prescriptive norms, but descriptive ones, relative to a "goal" of an organism. As such, biological dysfunctions do not necessarily call for medical, psychiatric, or psychotherapeutic treatment. In contrast to HDA*, BST* thus cannot make intelligible what it is about having a mental disorder that justifies certain normative consequences. BST* cannot make intelligible (1) why having a mental disorder gives the affected individual a *pro tanto* reason to seek psychiatric or psychotherapeutic treatment nor (2) why others have a *pro tanto* reason to help the affected individual in some way or to (partly) exempt or excuse them from certain social, legal, or moral obligations.

Here, a critic might object and argue that we, as a society, have an obligation to help the affected individual to return to a condition in which all their mechanisms perform their PBFs or NPFs. For example, if an individual suffers from a psychosis due to a dysfunction of a neural mechanism, then we have the obligation to offer them an appropriate treatment (if available).

Prima facie, this is a plausible view. But what justifies this obligation? One might think that the obligation can be justified by reference to the fact that when a mechanism is not performing its PBF or NPF, it is behaving in a way that it *should not* behave. But this will not suffice; because the sense in which the token mechanism is not behaving in the way it "should" behave is, by itself, not a morally significant one. To argue that the presence of a biological dysfunction has normative consequences one would have to make an additional claim; for instance, that the presence of a biological dysfunction involves, generally, the presence of something that is in a morally significant sense "bad." Or in other words, we must make the additional claim that proper/statistically normal biological functioning is generally good or valuable.

Notes

1 See Schramme (2003, 2007, 2010), Ananth (2008), and Heinz (2014, 2017) for similar views. See Tsou (2021) for a definition of MENTAL DISORDER in biological terms (namely, as "harmful biological kinds") but without reference to biological functions.

2 Sometimes "natural function" is used instead of "biological function" (see, for example, Wakefield 1992a). However, to talk about "natural functions" is misleading. Natural functions are distinguished from other types of functions with respect to the type of object to which they are ascribed. A natural function is the proper function of a naturally occurring mechanism, as opposed to, say, the proper function of an artifact (or, more precisely, an artificial mechanism). Artificial and naturally occurring entities are usually distinguished according to whether they are human-made. For instance, a light-switch mechanism is an artificial mechanism because it is human-made, whereas the heart's blood-pumping mechanism is a naturally occurring mechanism because it is not human-made. However, not all naturally occurring mechanisms in this sense are ascribed proper functions (for example, rock falls). Generally, when we ascribe proper functions to naturally occurring mechanisms, we ascribe them only to those that involve parts and processes of some type of organism. Thus, it is more accurate to talk of "biological functions" (functions of living things under a biological description) than of "natural functions" in general.

3 Parts of this chapter draw on Dembić (2023).

4 For an introduction to mechanisms, see Glennan (2016). For a comprehensive overview, see Glennan and Illari (2017).

5 See Krickel (2018) for a discussion of the metaphysics of mechanisms. According to her, there are at least three notions of mechanism that go beyond the minimal characterization: (1) functional mechanisms (mechanisms that serve a biological function), (2) regular mechanisms (mechanisms that regularly produce a particular phenomenon), and (3) reversely regular mechanisms (mechanisms that regularly produce some phenomenon).

6 For an overview of the competing views of the proper relata of causation, see Ehring (2010).

7 Functions are ascribed not only to mechanisms but also to organs, traits, or other entities that are not causal sequences of events. Is this in conflict with the view that functions are *effects*? Not necessarily, because one might hold (a) a different view on the relata of causation or (b) that organs or other entities can have functions insofar as they participate in causal sequences of events.

8 This view was introduced by Wright (1973). For similar views, see Papineau (1987), Millikan (1984, 1989), Neander (1991), Griffiths (1993), Godfrey-Smith (1994), and Griffiths and Matthewson (2018).

9 See Millikan (1984) for a similar proposal. Wakefield's own characterization (1992a, 382) is imprecise because it does not distinguish between types and tokens.

10 For a discussion, see Faucher and Forest (2021, chapters 11 and 12).

11 For critiques, see, for instance, Sadler and Agich (1995), Murphy and Woolfolk (2000), Thornton (2000), Boorse (2011), Kingma (2013), and Faucher and Forest (2021). For replies, see, for instance, Faucher and Forest (2021).

12 Cooper (2021, 758) makes a similar point.

13 See Lilienfeld and Marino (1995), Richters and Hinshaw (1999), Woolfolk (1999), Bolton (2001), Murphy and Stich (2000), and Murphy and Woolfolk (2000) for different versions of this type of objection. For a similar objection in terms of "developmental mismatches," see Garson (2021). For a reply, see Wakefield (2021).

14 See Schwartz (2007, 370) for a similar point concerning the problem of drawing the line between disorder and non-disorder.

15 The case might be different for DISEASE or BODILY DISORDER; Griffiths and Matthewson (2018) argue for an explication of DISEASE in terms of PBFs.

16 Boorse identifies "internal parts or processes" as the bearers of functions. For brevity, I shall use "mechanism" to denote the bearer of functions (see Section 3.1).

17 I follow Boorse in using the terms "normal" and "typical" in a statistical sense.

18 See Garson and Piccinini (2014) for a similar view.

19 Boorse uses the terms "readiness," "ability," and "disposition" interchangeably. In the philosophical literature, "readiness" is not a commonly used term and abilities are generally ascribed to agents performing actions rather than to parts of organisms. I shall therefore use "disposition."

20 See Keil (2007) for a more general discussion of the teleology problem in biology.

21 Boorse's view is in the tradition of Cummins' (1975) "containing system analysis" of FUNCTION.

22 Boorse's conception of FUNCTION applies to both organisms and artifacts (insofar as they are goal-directed systems).

23 Criticisms can be found in Engelhardt (1975, 1986), Margolis (1976), Mischel (1977), Whitbeck (1978), Agich (1983), Brown (1985), Lavin (1985), Hare (1986), Wulff, Pedersen, and Rosenberg(1986), Reznek (1987), Scadding (1988), van der Steen and Thung (1988), Fulford (1989), Amundson (2000), DeVito (2000), Nordenfelt (2001), Cooper (2002), Murphy (2006), Kingma (2007, 2010, 2013), Schwartz (2007), Ananth (2008), and Ereshefsky (2009), Giroux (2009), Hamilton (2010), Hausman (2011, 2012), Garson and Piccinini (2014), Heinz (2014), and Griffiths and Matthewson (2018). For replies and amendments, see Boorse (1997, 2014) and Hausman (2014).

24 Tsou (2021, 31) references Maung (2016) and Stegenga (2018, Chapter 4).

25 Bingham and Banner (2014) argue that the exclusion of homosexuality should serve as a test case for definitions of "mental disorder."

References

Agich, George J. 1983. "Disease and Value: A Rejection of the Value-Neutrality Thesis." *Theoretical Medicine* 4: 27–41.

Amundson, Ron. 2000. "Against Normal Function." *Studies in History and Philosophy of Science Part C: Studies in History and Philosophy of Biological and Biomedical Sciences* 31 (1): 33–53.

Ananth, Mahesh. 2008. *In Defense of an Evolutionary Concept of Health.* Aldershot: Ashgate.

Bechtel, William. 2008. "Mechanisms in Cognitive Psychology: What Are the Operations?" *Philosophy of Science* 75 (5): 983–994.

Bingham, Rachel, and Natalie Banner. 2014. "The Definition of Mental Disorder: Evolving but Dysfunctional?" *Journal of Medical Ethics* 40 (8): 537–542.

Bolton, Derek. 2001. "Problems in the Definition of 'Mental Disorder.'" *The Philosophical Quarterly* 51 (203): 182–199.

Boorse, Christopher. 1975. "On the Distinction between Disease and Illness." *Philosophy and Public Affairs* 5 (1): 49–68.

———. 1976a. "What a Theory of Mental Health Should Be." *Journal for the Theory of Social Behaviour* 6 (1): 61–84.

———. 1976b. "Wright on Functions." *Philosophical Review* 85 (1): 70–86.

———. 1977. "Health as a Theoretical Concept." *Philosophy of Science* 44 (4): 542–573.

———. 1997. "A Rebuttal on Health," In *What Is Disease?*, edited by James M. Humber and Robert F. Almeder, 1–134. New Jersey: Humana Press.

———. 2002. "A Rebuttal on Functions." In *Functions: New Essays in the Philosophy of Psychology and Biology*, edited by André Ariew, Robert C. Cummins, and Mark Perlman, 63–112. Oxford: Oxford University Press.

———. 2011. "Concepts of Health and Disease." In *Philosophy of Medicine*, edited by Fred Gifford, 13–64. Munich: Elsevier.

———. 2014. "A Second Rebuttal on Health." *Journal of Medicine and Philosophy* 39 (6): 683–724.

Brown, W. Miller. 1985. "On Defining 'Disease.'" *Journal of Medicine and Philosophy* 10: 311–328.

Cooper, Rachel. 2002. "Disease." *Studies in History and Philosophy of Science* 33 (2): 263–282.

———. 2005. *Classifying Madness: A Philosophical Examination of the Diagnostic and Statistical Manual of Mental Disorders*. Dordrecht: Springer.

———. 2007. *Psychiatry and Philosophy of Science*. Durham: Acumen.

———. 2021. "On Harm." In *Defining Mental Disorder: Jerome Wakefield and his Critics*, edited by Luc Faucher and Denis Forest, chapter 26. Cambridge, MA: MIT Press.

Craver, Carl F. 2007. *Explaining the Brain: Mechanisms and the Mosaic Unity of Neuroscience*. Oxford: Oxford University Press.

Cummins, Robert. 1975. "Functional Analysis." *Journal of Philosophy* 72 (20): 741–764.

Dawkins, Richard. 1976. *The Selfish Gene*. Oxford: Oxford University Press.

Dembić, Sanja. 2023. "Mental Disorder: An Ability-Based View." *Philosophy and the Mind Sciences* 4 (2): 1–28.

DeVito, Scott. 2000. "On the Value-Neutrality of the Concepts of Health and Disease: Unto the Breach Again." *Journal of Medicine and Philosophy* 25 (5): 539–567.

Ehring, Douglas. 2010. "Causal Relata." In *The Oxford Handbook of Causation*, edited by Helen Beebee, Christopher Hitchcock, and Peter Menzies, chapter 19. Oxford: Oxford University Press.

Engelhardt, H. Tristram Jr. 1975. "The Concepts of Health and Disease." In *Evaluation and Explanation in the Biomedical Sciences*, edited by H. Tristram Engelhardt Jr. and Stuart F. Spicker (1st edn), 125–141. Dordrecht: D. Reidel Publishing Company.

———. 1986. *The Foundations of Bioethics*. Oxford: Oxford University Press.

Ereshefsky, Marc. 2009. "Defining 'Health' and 'Disease.'" *Studies in History and Philosophy of Science* 40 (3): 221–227.

Faucher, Luc, and Denis Forest. 2021. *Defining Mental Disorder: Jerome Wakefield and His Critics*. Cambridge, MA: MIT Press.

Feit, Neil. 2017. "Harm and the Concept of Mental Disorder." *Theoretical Medicine and Bioethics* 38 (5): 367–385.

Fulford, William K. M. 1989. *Moral Theory and Medical Practice*. Cambridge: Cambridge University Press.

Garson, Justin. 2021. "The Developmental Plasticity Challenge to Wakefield's View." In *Defining Mental Disorder: Jerome Wakefield and His Critics*, edited by Luc Faucher and Denis Forest, chapter 16. Cambridge: MIT Press.

Garson, Justin, and Gualtiero Piccinini. 2014. "Functions Must Be Performed at Appropriate Rates in Appropriate Situations." *The British Journal for the Philosophy of Science* 65 (1): 1–20.

Giroux, Élodie. 2009. "Définir objectivement la santé: une évaluation du concept biostatistique de Boorse à partir de l'épidémiologie modern." *Revue Philosophique de la France et de l'Étranger* 134 (1): 35–58.

Glennan, Stuart. 1996. "Mechanisms and the Nature of Causation." *Erkenntnis* 44 (1): 49–71.

———. 2016. "Mechanisms and Mechanical Philosophy." In *The Oxford Handbook of Philosophy of Science*, edited by Paul Humphreys, 796–816. Oxford: Oxford University Press.

Glennan, Stuart, and Phyllis Illari. 2017. *The Routledge Handbook of Mechanisms and Mechanical Philosophy*. London: Routledge.

Griffiths, Paul E. 1993. "Functional Analysis and Proper Function." *British Journal for Philosophy of Science* 44: 409–422.

Griffiths, Paul E., and John Matthewson. 2018. "Evolution, Dysfunction, and Disease: A Reappraisal." *British Journal for Philosophy of Science* 69: 301–327.

Godfrey-Smith, Peter. 1994. "A Modern History Theory of Functions." *Noûs* 28: 344–362.

Gould, Stephen J., and Richard C. Lewontin. 1979. "The Spandrels of San Marco and the Panglossian Paradigm: A Critique of the Adaptionist Programme." *Proceedings of the Royal Society B: Biological Sciences* 205 (1161): 252–270.

Gould, Stephen J., and Elisabeth S. Vrba. 1982. "Exaptation: A Missing Term in the Science of Form." *Paleobiology* 8 (1): 4–15.

Hamilton, Richard P. 2010. "The Concept of Health: Beyond Normativism and Naturalism" *Journal of Evaluation in Clinical Practice* 16 (2): 323–329.

Hausman, Daniel M. 2011. "Is an Overdose of Paracetamol Bad for One's Health?" *The British Journal for the Philosophy of Science* 62: 657–668.

———. 2012. "Health, Naturalism, and Functional Efficiency." *Philosophy of Science* 79: 519–541.

———. 2014. "Health and Functional Efficiency." *Journal of Medicine and Philosophy* 39: 634–647.

Hare, Richard M. 1986. "Health." *Journal of Medical Ethics* 12 (4): 174–181.

Heinz, Andreas. 2014. *Der Begriff der psychischen Krankheit*. Berlin: Suhrkamp.

———. 2017. *A New Understanding of Mental Disorders: Computational Models for Dimensional Psychiatry*. Cambridge, MA: MIT Press.

Hempel, Carl G., and Paul Oppenheim. 1948. "Studies in the Logic of Explanation." *Philosophy of Science* 15 (2): 135–175.

Kingma, Elselijn. 2007. "What Is It to Be Healthy?" *Analysis* 67 (2): 128–133.

———. 2010. "Paracetamol, Poison, and Polio: Why Boorse's Account of Function Fails to Distinguish Health and Disease." *The British Journal for the Philosophy of Science* 61 (2): 261–264.

———. 2013. "Naturalist Accounts of Mental Disorder." In *The Oxford Handbook of Philosophy and Psychiatry*, edited by William K. M. Fulford, Martin Davies, Richard Gipps, George Graham, John Sadler, Giovanni Stanghellini, and Tim Thornton, 363–384. Oxford: Oxford University Press.

Keil, Geert. 2007. "Biologische Funktionen und das Teleologieproblem." In *Naturalismus als Paradigma. Wie weit reicht die naturwissenschaftliche Erklärung des Menschen?*, edited by Ludger Honnefelder and Matthias C. Schmidt, 76–85. Berlin: Berlin University Press.

Kraemer, Daniel M. 2013. "Statistical Theories of Functions and the Problem of Epidemic Disease." *Biology and Philosophy* 28: 423–438.

Krickel, Beate. 2018. *The Mechanical World: The Metaphysical Commitments of the New Mechanistic Approach*. Basel: Springer International Publishing.

Lavin, Michael. 1985. "Doctors, Psychiatrists, and Disease." *Social Science and Medicine* 20 (5): 535–543.

Lilienfeld, Scott O., and Lori Marino. 1995. "Mental Disorder as a Roschian Concept: A Critique of Wakefield's 'Harmful Dysfunction' Analysis." *Journal of Abnormal Psychology* 104 (3): 411–420.

Machamer, Peter K., Lindley Darden, and Carl F. Craver. 2000. "Thinking About Mechanisms." *Philosophy of Science* 67 (1): 1–25.

Margolis, Joseph. 1976. "The Concept of Disease." *Journal of Medicine and Philosophy* 1 (3): 238–255.

Maung, Hane H. 2016. "Diagnosis and Causal Explanation in Psychiatry." *Studies in History and Philosophy of Biological and Biomedical Sciences* 60: 15–24.

Melander, Peter. 1997. *Analyzing Functions: An Essay on a Fundamental Notion in Biology*. Stockholm: Almqvist and Wiksell.

Millikan, Ruth G. 1984. *Language, Thought and Other Biological Categories: New Foundations for Realism*. Cambridge, MA: MIT Press.

———. 1989. "In Defense of Proper Functions." *Philosophy of Science* 56: 288–302.

Mischel, Theodore. 1977. "The Concept of Mental Health and Disease: An Analysis of the Controversy between Behavioral and Psychodynamic Approaches." *Journal of Medicine and Philosophy* 2 (3): 197–219.

Murphy, Dominic. 2006. *Psychiatry in the Scientific Image*. Cambridge, MA: MIT Press.

———. 2020. "Concepts of Disease and Health". In *Stanford Encyclopedia of Philosophy*, edited by Edward N. Zalta, (Fall 2020 ed.) https://plato.stanford.edu/archives/fall2020/entries/psychiatry/.

Murphy, Dominic, and Stephen Stich. 2000. "Darwin in the Madhouse: Evolutionary Psychology and the Classification of Mental Disorders." In *Evolution and the Human Mind: Modularity, Language and Meta-Cognition*, edited by Peter Carruthers and Andrew Chamberlain, 62–92. Cambridge: Cambridge University Press.

Murphy, Dominic and Robert L. Woolfolk. 2000. "Conceptual Analysis Versus Scientific Understanding: An Assessment of Wakefield's Folk Psychiatry." *Philosophy, Psychiatry, and Psychology* 7 (4): 271–293.

Nagel, Ernest. 1961. *The Structure of Science: Problems in the Logic of Scientific Explanation*. New York: Harcourt, Brace and World.

Neander, Karen. 1991. "Functions as Selected Effects: The Conceptual Analyst's Defense." *Philosophy of Science* 58 (2): 168–184.

Nordenfelt, Lennart. 2001. *Health, Science, and Ordinary Language*. New York: Rodopi.

———. 2003. "On the Evolutionary Concept of Health: Health as a Natural Function," In *Dimensions of Health and Health Promotion*, edited by Lennart Nordenfelt and Per-Erik Liss, 37–53. Amsterdam: Rodopi.

Papineau, David. 1987. *Reality and Representation*. New York: Blackwell.

Reznek, Lawrie. 1987. *The Nature of Disease*. London: Routledge.

Richters, John E., and Stephen P. Hinshaw. 1999. "The Abduction of Disorder in Psychiatry." *Journal of Abnormal Psychology* 108 (3): 438–445.

Sadler, John Z., and George J. Agich. 1995. "Diseases, Functions, Values, and Psychiatric Classification." *Philosophy, Psychiatry, and Psychology* 2 (3): 219–231.

Salmon, Wesley C. 1984. *Scientific Explanation and the Causal Structure of the World*. Princeton: Princeton University Press.

Scadding, John G. 1988. "Health and Disease: What Can Medicine Do for Philosophy?" *Journal of Medical Ethics* 14 (3): 118–124.

Schramme, Thomas. 2003. *Psychische Krankheiten aus philosophischer Sicht*. Giessen: Psychosozial-Verlag.

———. 2007. "A Qualified Defense of a Naturalist Theory of Health." *Medicine, Health Care and Philosophy* 10 (1): 11–17.

———. 2010. "Can We Define Mental Disorder by Using the Criterion of Mental Dysfunction?" *Theoretical Medicine and Bioethics* 31 (1): 35–47.

Schwartz, Peter H. 2007. "Defining Dysfunction: Natural Selection, Design, and Drawing a Line." *Philosophy of Science* 74 (3): 364–385.

Sommerhoff, Gerd. 1950. *Analytical Biology*. Oxford: Oxford University Press.

———. 1959. "The Abstract Characteristics of Living Organisms." In *Systems Thinking*, edited by Frederick E. Emery, 147–202. London: Harmondsworth.

Stegenga, Jacob. 2018. *Medical Nihilism*. Oxford: Oxford University Press.

Thornton, Tim. 2000. "Mental Illness and Reductionism: Can Functions Be Naturalized?" *Philosophy, Psychiatry, and Psychology* 7 (1): 67–76.

Tsou, Jonathan Y. 2021. *Philosophy of Psychiatry*. Cambridge: Cambridge University Press.

van der Steen, Wim J., and Paul J. Thung. 1988. *Faces of Medicine: A Philosophical Study*. Dordrecht: Kluwer.

Wakefield, Jerome C. 1992a. "The Concept of Mental Disorder. On the Boundary between Biological Facts and Social Values." *American Psychologist* 47 (3): 373–388.

———. 1992b. "Disorder as Harmful Dysfunction: A Conceptual Critique of DSM-III-R's Definition of Mental Disorder." *Psychological Review* 99 (2): 232–247.

———. 1999. "Evolutionary versus Prototype Analyses of the Concept of Disorder." *Journal of Abnormal Psychology* 108: 374–399.

———. 2000. "Spandrels, Vestigial Organs, and Such: Reply to Murphy and Woolfolk's 'the Harmful Dysfunction Analysis of Mental Disorder.'" *Philosophy, Psychiatry, and Psychology* 7 (4): 253–269.

———. 2006. "What Makes a Mental Disorder Mental?" *Philosophy, Psychiatry, and Psychology* 13 (2): 123–131.

———. 2013. "Addiction, the Concept of Disorder, and Pathways to Harm: Comment on Levy." *Frontiers in Psychiatry* 4 (34): 1–2.

———. 2014. "The Biostatistical Theory versus the Harmful Dysfunction Analysis, Part 1: Is Part-Dysfunction a Sufficient Condition for Medical Disorder?" *Journal of Medicine and Philosophy* 39 (6): 648–682.

———. 2021. "Is the Harmful Dysfunction Analysis Descriptive or Stipulative, and Is the HDA or BST the Better Naturalist Account of Dysfunction? Reply to Maël Lemoine." In *Defining Mental Disorder: Jerome Wakefield and his Critics*, edited by Luc Faucher and Denis Forest, chapters 12 and 17. Cambridge, MA: MIT Press.

Whitbeck, Caroline. 1978. "Four Basic Concepts of Medical Science." In *PSA 1978*, edited by Peter D. Asquith and Ian Hacking, 210–222. East Lansing: Philosophy of Science Association.

Woolfolk, Robert L. 1999. "Malfunction and Mental Illness." *The Monist* 82 (4): 658–670.

Wolf, Susan. 2010. *Meaning in Life and Why It Matters*. Princeton: Princeton University Press.

Wright, Larry. 1973. "Functions." *Philosophical Review* 82 (2): 139–168.

Wulff, Henrik R., Stig A. Pedersen, and Raben Rosenberg. 1986. *Philosophy of Medicine: An Introduction*. Oxford: Blackwell Scientific Publications.

4 The Rehability View

In this chapter, I will present the view that I want to defend. I call this the Rehability View (RHA) because it explicates MENTAL DISORDER in terms of REASONS, HARM, and ABILITY. The chapter is structured as follows. In Section 4.1, I introduce and motivate RHA. In Sections 4.2–4.4, I elaborate on the concepts ABILITY, REASONS, and HARM, respectively. In Section 4.5, I develop and illustrate RHA by way of a case study of anxiety disorder. In Section 4.6, I present the full version of RHA.[1]

4.1 Introducing the Rehability View

To introduce RHA, I will present a version of the RHA that is confined to the clearest (types of) cases that should fall under MENTAL DISORDER.[2] For the purposes specified in Section 1.2, I propose the following explication of MENTAL DISORDER.

RHA An individual S has a mental disorder if and only if

  i   S does not have the *ability* to respond adequately to some of their available (apparent) *reasons* for (or against) some of their reason-sensitive attitudes or actions and
  ii S is *harmed* by their condition C.[3]

In the course of this chapter, I will explain what exactly is meant by this explication and elaborate on the relevant concepts—ABILITY, REASONS, and HARM—in turn. In doing so, I will gradually introduce more details and present the full version of RHA in Section 4.6. I therefore ask the reader for patience.

RHA is based on the following basic ideas:

1 Having a mental disorder is a matter of not having (or: lacking) the ability to φ.[4]
2 Mental disorder involves φ-ings that are sensitive to reasons.

DOI: 10.4324/9781003367840-5

3 S's condition C is worthy of psychiatric or psychotherapeutic concern
only if S is harmed by C.

When we ascribe a mental disorder to an individual, we are basically claiming that they "cannot" (in the relevant sense) do something, where the
"something" they "cannot" do involves attitudes or actions that are sensitive to reasons (at least in the clearest cases of mental disorder). There are
reasons for (or against) both attitudes (for example, beliefs and emotions)
and actions. Generally, to respond to one's available (apparent) reasons for
attitude A (or action φ) is to form attitude A (or to φ or intend to φ).[5] Likewise, to respond to one's available (apparent) reasons against attitude A (or
action φ) is to omit forming attitude A (or to omit φ-ing or intending to φ).

Recall that RHA is an explication of MENTAL DISORDER for both theoretical and practical purposes (see Section 1.2). To obtain an explication of
MENTAL DISORDER for theoretical purposes only, I propose that we omit
condition (2), which states that it is necessary for S to be harmed by C (I
return to this issue in Section 5.5).

Before describing RHA in some detail, let me note an important caveat,
make two clarifications, and motivate the view.

Caveat. We should not confuse an inability to φ with an inability to *learn*
to φ. The ability to learn to φ is a second-order ability: the ability to ac-
quire the ability to φ. That S does not have the first-order ability to φ does
not entail that S does not have the second-order ability to learn to φ (or in
other words: the potential to φ). I may currently lack the ability to do 75
pull-ups, but this does not imply that I do not have the potential to do so.
Individuals may also lose abilities. I used to be able to speak French quite
well, but today *pas tellement*.

This is important to keep in mind because it clarifies that RHA does not
imply that an individual with a mental disorder cannot overcome their mental disorder (possibly even on their own). The ability to overcome one's mental disorder is the ability to learn the ability one lacks when one has a mental
disorder. As such, it is a second-order ability. RHA, however, ascribes a
first-order inability and as we have seen, an ascription of a first-order inability does not imply an ascription of a second-order inability.

Clarification (1). RHA's core idea—that having a mental disorder is a matter of not having a certain ability to φ—needs to be relativized. Obviously,
not every inability marks a disorder. Humans are not able to fly (without
technical equipment), but this does not constitute a bodily disorder. Humans are also not able to read and memorize a novel in two seconds, but
this does not constitute a mental disorder. This suggests that the ability-
condition must be relativized to what humans *in general* can do.

This has, at least, two consequences. First, any conception of MENTAL DISORDER that refers to ABILITIES must specify what "in general" means. Second, any such view must be backed by an account of which types of abilities humans generally have. The former is a task for philosophers, while the latter is a task for psychologists (the former being a conceptual question and the latter being an empirical question). RHA is neutral with respect to (1) how exactly generic statements should be understood and (2) what exactly humans' psychological structure(s) look like. This is not a shortfall, but rather a strength of the view. One can endorse RHA without having to endorse any specific semantic theory of generic statements or any specific psychological theory about humans. This is not to say that different theories may not yield that different phenomena fall under MENTAL DISORDER. However, my task is to explicate MENTAL DISORDER, and not to provide a list of mental disorders.

Nevertheless, two points are important for any such theory.

First, it is clear that human abilities generally vary with developmental stage (which does not necessarily equate to age). What babies can do is mostly different from what adults can do. Likewise, what counts as a disorder is relative to an individual's developmental stage. It is not necessarily a disorder for a baby to lack some ability that an adult has (for example, speaking in full sentences).

Second, statements about what humans can generally do will be *generic* ones, such as "humans have 32 teeth." Generic statements are generalizations. But, unlike quantified statements (for example, "all humans have 32 teeth"), they do not inform us about how many members of the reference class have the stated property. Thus, what humans (at a certain developmental stage) can generally do does not equate to those abilities that it is statistically normal for them to have. Similarly, the generic statement "humans have 32 teeth" is true, even if it is probably not statistically normal for humans to have 32 teeth.

It is difficult to semantically analyze generic statements (under which conditions is it true to claim that humans have 32 teeth?). There is ongoing debate on this issue, and any comprehensive view of mental disorder that depends on generic statements will have to say something about it.[6] Thus, generic statements pose a challenge not only for RHA. Any theory of mental (or bodily) disorder will face this challenge because it will have to rely on the insights from psychology (or physiology), and making generalizations is exactly what special scientists (psychologists or physiologists) are trying to do.[7] Different semantic theories of generic statements might yield different verdicts on which abilities humans generally have. But they cannot diverge to a great extent while all being true. A glimpse at psychology textbooks reveals that we have a firm grasp on which abilities humans generally have.

Clarification (2). Not all abilities that humans generally have are relevant to assessing their health. Humans can generally roll their tongues, but lacking this ability does not mark a disorder.[8] Why not? A first line of reasoning is that it is because such an ability is not relevant to the survival of humans. However, health and disorder are intimately related to survival. It is conceptually impossible for an individual to be both dead and completely healthy. A second line of reasoning—one that I prefer—is that lacking the ability to role one's tongue does not mark a disorder because it is an ability that is not relevant to the purposes for which we should use the concept DISORDER.[9] According to the second line of reasoning, we need to restrict the abilities in light of the broader theoretical framework which is provided by the method of explication (see Chapter 1).

RHA proposes that in the field of mental disorder only those abilities that, when diminished, present a harm to their bearer are relevant. In addition, HARM should be understood more broadly than "detrimental to one's survival." On the view I propose, HARM should be understood as "being detrimental to living a life that is (sufficiently) worth living for the individual who lives it" (see Section 4.4.) The reasoning behind this view is the following. One purpose for which we use the concept MENTAL DISORDER is to help us determine who should seek psychiatric or psychotherapeutic treatment (see Section 1.3). More specifically, an individual with a mental disorder has a *pro tanto* reason to seek psychiatric or psychotherapeutic treatment (if available). Now, an individual does not only have such a reason in case their life is at stake but also when they are living a life that is, for them, not a life (sufficiently) worth living. In short, when assessing mental disorder, we care about more than mere survival, or so I claim.

In sum, I propose that only those abilities are relevant in the field of mental disorder that meet the following two conditions:

1 they are abilities that humans generally have, and
2 they are abilities that, when diminished, present a harm to their bearer.

Let me now motivate the three basic ideas behind RHA.

Inability. To motivate the first idea—that mental disorders involve inabilities of some sort—imagine the following scenarios:

a Saying "just relax" to an individual with an anxiety disorder.
b Saying "just cheer up" to an individual with a major depressive disorder.
c Saying "just stop thinking that someone is following you" to an individual with a delusional disorder.
d Saying "just stop using" to an individual with an addictive disorder.

Such responses seem to miss the point. An individual with an anxiety disorder precisely cannot stop experiencing fear in certain situations, an individual with a major depressive disorder precisely cannot stop feeling depressed, and so on. If having the ability to φ is a necessary condition for being obliged to φ, then demanding that an individual φ when they "cannot" do so is inadequate. One purpose of this chapter is to specify the exact sense in which an individual with a mental disorder "cannot" φ.

Sensitivity to Reasons. To motivate the second idea—that mental disorder involves φ-ing that are sensitive to reasons—consider the difference between delusion and diabetes. The *DSM-5* characterizes delusions as "fixed beliefs that are not amenable to change in light of conflicting evidence" (APA 2013, 87). To illustrate this, consider Bill, an individual suffering from schizophrenia. One night, while watching television, Bill suddenly came to believe that

> a group of conspirators had secretly produced and distributed a documentary about his homosexual experiences. Several of his high school friends and a few distant relatives had presumably used hidden cameras and microphones to record each of his sexual encounters with other men. Bill believed that the film had grossed over $50 million at the box office and that this money had been sent to the Irish Republican Army to buy arms and ammunition. He therefore held himself responsible for the deaths of dozens of people who had died as the result of several recent bombings in Ireland.
>
> (Oltmanns et al. 2012, 131)

Whatever phenomena count as "delusional" can neither be "picked out" nor understood without referring to certain types of mental states (or attitudes) that are sensitive to reasons. At a minimum, delusions are beliefs (or belief-like cognitive states) that are, in some sense, "disordered" with respect to the (apparent) reasons available to an individual. Bill's beliefs are not merely undesirable for him. Rather, something is amiss with his available (apparent) reasons for his beliefs.

By contrast, consider diabetes. Diabetes is a group of metabolic diseases where individuals have high blood glucose because insulin production is inadequate, because body cells do not respond properly to insulin, or both. Although the production of insulin can be "adequate" or "inadequate" and body cells can respond "properly" or "improperly," they are not inadequate or improper responses to available reasons.[10] We can explain why body cells do not respond properly to insulin by referring to a certain causal process. But it makes no sense to cite something as a reason *for* (or *against*) body cells responding improperly to insulin. However, we can (1) explain why an individual has a certain belief p by referring to a certain causal process and (2) ask them for their reasons for or against p.

Harm. To motivate the third idea—that S's condition C is worthy of psychiatric or psychotherapeutic concern only if S is harmed by C—consider cases of what we may call "harmless disorders." Small paper cuts are typically harmless pathological bodily conditions. This is why we tell children not to worry about them. Cases like this show that "harmless bodily disorder" is not an oxymoron. Cases of harmless disorder can also be found in the mental realm. Consider an individual with an excessive fear of spiders who lives in a spider-free environment. In this context, their condition is harmless (assuming that they are not preoccupied with their fear when spiders are absent). It might still make sense, though, to claim that they have a mental disorder (namely a specific phobia related to spiders). However, it is a disorder that the affected individual does not need to worry about. The condition does not provide them with a *pro tanto* reason to seek psychiatric or psychotherapeutic treatment (which is why on the view I propose "harmless disorders" are only "disorders" in a purely theoretical sense). We do not and (unless there are mitigating reasons) should not care too much about harmless disorders. But we do and should care about disorders that are harmful to their bearers.

These remarks on motivation do not constitute a full defense of RHA. They are supposed to make the basic ideas *prima facie* plausible. I shall defend RHA in Chapter 5. Before doing so, let me explicate it in some more detail.

4.2 Abilities

The core idea behind RHA is that having a mental disorder is a matter of not having the ability to φ. I start elaborating on this idea by making four points related to abilities quite generally.[11]

First, having an ability to φ is a modal property possessed by an agent, that is, an individual who has the capacity for action. It relates an individual to what they *can* or *could* do and not necessarily to what they actually do.[12] For an individual to have the ability to φ, it is not necessary that they ever actually φ. I have the ability to dress up like a zombie and participate in a "zombie run," but chances are high that I will never do so. In other words, the ability to φ can be instantiated in an individual without them ever actually exercising it. Nevertheless, for the individual to have the ability to φ, it must at least be possible for them to φ.

Second, abilities relate an individual to an action or to some non-agentive process.[13] There are then agentive and non-agentive abilities. A human being (typically) has the ability to sing but also the ability to digest food. The ability to sing is agentive because singing is an action; the ability to digest food is non-agentive because digestion is not an action.

Third, having an ability is typically not an all-or-nothing matter. It is a matter of degree. I can dance better now than I did before because I have had several years of dancing lessons, but Mikhail Baryshnikov is still a better dancer than I am. We can compare an individual's abilities over time or compare the abilities of different individuals (at the same time or over time). Theoretically, it is possible to hierarchically arrange individuals' abilities along a continuum.

Although abilities come in degrees, we often make categorical ascriptions. That is, we often claim that an individual "has" or "does not have" some ability *simpliciter*. Or, we often ask whether an individual has some ability or not, thereby expecting a yes-or-no answer. In many cases in which we say that an individual "does not have" some ability, we do not mean that they have zero degrees of that ability. If I am asked "can you sing?" at an opera casting, then it would be misleading of me to answer "yes." But, of course, my answer does not imply that I cannot sing *at all*. What I meant was that I cannot sing *well enough* to perform in an opera. To account for this, we should understand the locution "S does not have the ability to φ" as "S's ability to φ is not sufficiently high" (alternatively, "S does not have the ability to φ to a sufficient degree").

This specification leads to a further question. What fixes the degree above which an ability counts as "sufficient"? In other words, what determines the threshold on the scale of some ability above which ascriptions of that ability apply categorically? One solution is to appeal to the ascriber context (the context in which the ascription is made), more specifically, to the standards that obtain in a given ascriber context (see Jaster 2020).[14] On this view, different standards will obtain in different practical contexts. Which standards obtain, in turn, depends on the interests of the relevant individuals or the *purposes* for which they make the ability ascriptions in the first place. For example, in the context of an opera casting, the degree of singing ability that counts as "sufficient" will be higher than the one in a karaoke bar.

Fourth, abilities are always had "in view of" some facts (see Kratzer 1977). Consider a professional swimmer with a broken arm. Can they swim? In some sense, they can (they are a professional swimmer), but, in another sense, they cannot (they have a broken arm, after all). In the literature, this is typically expressed by saying that they have the "general," but not the "specific," ability to swim (see Honoré 1964 and Mele 2003). We can distinguish between these two senses by specifying the facts in view of which we evaluate whether they can swim or not. In view of the fact that they are a professional swimmer it is true that they can swim. But, in view of the fact that they currently have a broken arm, it is true that they cannot swim. In the first sense, but not the second sense, we abstract away from the fact that they currently have a broken arm.

This view traces back to Angelika Kratzer's (1977) modal semantics. On Kratzer's (1977, 342) view, there is no absolute sense of "can." Rather, "S can φ" should be understood as "S can, in view of F, φ," where F specifies a contextually selected set of facts in view of which the ability to φ is ascribed.[15] On this view, there are only relative senses of "can." An individual S "can" (or "cannot") φ depending on which facts are relevant to the context in which we are interested in knowing whether S "can" φ. So, when evaluating whether S has the ability to φ, we must begin by specifying which facts are relevant to the context in which we are interested in knowing whether S has the ability to φ.

Given the aforementioned, we must specify RHA's core idea—that mental disorders involve inabilities of some sort—in terms of the following questions:

1 What types of φ-ings are involved in mental disorder?
2 What determines the threshold of inability in mental disorder?
3 In view of which facts does an individual with a mental disorder not have a certain ability to φ?

Types of φ-ings. In mental disorder, the relevant φ-ings might be either agentive or non-agentive. Using some drug is typically an action, but feeling sad or depressed is not. Emotions and moods are states, events, or processes that happen to us.[16] They are not something we do, and, *a fortiori*, not something that we do intentionally. In developing RHA, the difference between agentive and non-agentive φ-ings must be taken into account.

Threshold. Here, the question is "for which purpose(s) will an individual's abilities to respond adequately to their available (apparent) reasons have to be good enough for the individual to *not* have a mental disorder?" My general (and underspecified) answer is this: to live a life that is (sufficiently) worth living for the individual who lives it (see Section 4.4). When it comes to health, survival seems to be an overly modest goal, and living the ideally good life (whatever that is) seems to be an overly ambitious one.

Where exactly will the threshold be? Roughly, the view I propose is that the mental health-relevant ability needs to be so low that the affected individuals are typically harmed by it in some relevant respect (see Section 4.4). More specifically, I propose that to determine the threshold in an individual case, we have to compare S's ability to φ to the abilities to φ of the individuals in a relevant comparison class. First, we have to identify the relevant comparison class (along dimensions such as developmental stage, cultural context, and so forth). Second, we have to identify at which point the abilities to φ of the individuals in the relevant comparison are so low that these individuals are, on average, harmed by their condition in some relevant respect. Third, we have to determine whether S's degree of ability to φ is equal to or below that threshold.

Relevant Facts. I propose that the facts we need to consider when evaluating whether an individual has a mental disorder are, at a minimum, those about their *mental constitution*. Roughly, an individual's mental constitution comprises their relatively stable mental properties. These include their general beliefs, emotions, personality traits, attribution styles, and so on. Why these properties? When ascribing a mental disorder to an individual, we are not interested in knowing what they can do given every one of their actual mental states at the time of diagnosis. For instance, to determine whether an individual has a major depressive disorder, we should not consider the brief depressiveness they feel after reading *All Quiet on the Western Front*. In light of that mental state, an evaluation might yield that they have a depressive disorder when they do not. In ascribing a mental disorder, we ascribe an inability in a more general sense. More specifically, for the purposes of diagnosis, we are interested in knowing what this particular individual can do (and not what they could do if they were a different person). So, we should consider all the relatively stable mental properties that make up their individuality at the time of the diagnosis. Psychology and the closely related sciences will have to specify which types of stable mental properties there are and which of them are relevant for which types of mental disorders.

Having a mental disorder is not merely a matter of lacking the ability to φ in view of one's mental constitution. Certain facts that are external to an individual must also be taken into account. Why? For one, though abilities are properties of individuals, their *exercise* typically depends on the presence of certain extrinsic circumstances. For instance, to exercise the ability to ride a bicycle, the individual will have to have access to a bicycle. Simon Kittle calls "the set of conditions which are prerequisites for the very possibility of performing the type of action in question the *action-realisation conditions*" (2015, 3019). Some of these action-realization conditions are external circumstances. For another, in many contexts, we are interested in knowing whether an individual has the ability to φ in our actual world (in contrast to a possible world in which, for example, all kinds of miracles happen). For example, when we evaluate whether someone has the ability to ride a bicycle, we usually mean: in this world. Thus, in these contexts, we hold the actual laws of nature fixed and exclude all possible worlds in which all kinds of miracles happen.[17]

When it comes to mental disorder, the relevant external circumstances must be restricted even further. I propose that the ones that matter for mental disorder are roughly all external circumstances in an individual's life that they cannot easily change. I shall call these the individual's "life circumstances." This is, however, imprecise and will need to be specified further. Here, RHA can incorporate some psychiatry-critical ideas, such as the idea that mental disorder depends (at least in part) on sociocultural structures, power relations, and structural barriers.[18] This is because sociocultural structures are also part of the external circumstances that an individual cannot easily change.

In sum, on RHA, having a mental disorder is a matter of lacking the ability to φ in view of one's mental constitution and one's life circumstances, where the former comprises one's relatively stable mental properties and the latter the relatively stable external circumstances of one's life. Recognizing that the abilities relevant to mental disorder are always relative to certain external circumstances has consequences for therapy. For example, it makes it intelligible that, in some cases, it is possible to enable an individual with a mental disorder by changing their external circumstances.[19]

Let me now elaborate on what exactly it is to have an ability. I shall use Romy Jaster's (2020) "Success View" of abilities to spell out RHA in more detail. This is because Jaster's view can account for those features of abilities required for explicating MENTAL DISORDER.[20]

Here is Jaster's (2020, 98 and 159) (paraphrased) view of agentive abilities:

SUCCESS$_{AA}$ S has an agentive ability to perform an action φ if and only if S φs in a sufficiently high proportion of the relevant possible situations in which S intends to φ (where the set of the relevant possible situations will vary across ascriber contexts).

A darts player has the ability to hit the bull's-eye if and only if they hit it in a sufficiently high proportion of the relevant possible situations in which they intend to hit it. What counts for having an ability is a certain ratio. In the agentive case, it is the ratio of (a) the relevant possible intention situations in which the individual φs to (b) the totality of all relevant possible situations in which the individual intends to φ. Jaster calls this an individual's "modal success rate" (2020, 96). On this view, to have an ability is to exhibit a certain modal behavioral pattern. *Ceteris paribus*, the higher the modal success rate, the higher the degree of an ability will be. What if there is no relevant intentional situation to begin with? Then, the modal success rate will be unspecified or zero. In these cases, SUCCESS$_{AA}$ yields that the individual does not have the ability to φ because the relevant ratio would not be sufficiently high. Note that an individual's modal success rate should not be conflated with their "actual track record" (that is, the ratio of success cases among *actual* intention situations). An individual's track record only plays a heuristic role. A good track record gives us reason to believe that the individual has the ability to φ.

On Jaster's analysis, those facts in view of which an ability is ascribed determine the "relevant possible situations." The relevant possible situations are those situations in which the facts in view of which we are interested in knowing whether S has the ability to φ are held fixed. All other facts are varied. Let us say that we want to know whether a darts player has the ability to hit the bull's-eye in view of having a broken arm. We can evaluate their modal success rate among the possible intention situations in which they have a broken arm (we can though vary whether they are in a bar or some other place). Which possible situations are relevant varies with the purposes for which we want to know whether S has the ability to φ.

For Jaster, "intention" has a very specific reading. It is "an *action-initiating* propositional attitude in the sense that it is part of its causal role that it will typically initiate behavioral episodes corresponding to its content" (Jaster 2020, 101). By contrast, intentions to φ in the future (say, to stop smoking next year) are not action-initiating intentions. On Jaster's view, it does not count against S's ability to φ if S intends to φ in the future but does not φ when the time comes. This is because there may be an alternative explanation for why S did not φ; they may simply have given up their intention.

Jaster does not seem to think that there are alternative explanations in cases in which S intends to φ now but does not φ. I do not think that this is correct. There are still some alternative explanations left. Perhaps, S has the ability to φ, but simply

1 did not put enough effort in trying to φ;
2 made an inadvertent mistake when φ-ing; or
3 some accidental occurrence came between S initiating the action and the action's completion.

For instance, a dancer may have the ability to do a pirouette but fail to perform one when intending to do so. Possible explanations are (1) the dancer was not sufficiently focused or was not putting sufficient energy into their performance, (2) they accidentally stepped in the wrong way, or (3) someone bumped into them while they were performing the pirouette. This suggests that, although succeeding to φ counts in favor of having the ability to φ, *not* succeeding to φ (when intending to do so) does not necessarily count in favor of *not* having the ability to φ.

One way of dealing with this problem would be to simply exclude these kinds of situations when evaluating an individual's ability. That is, we could restrict the relevant possible situations to those in which the aforementioned scenarios—(1), (2), and (3)—do not occur. Another solution might lie in the Success View itself. What matters for having the ability to φ, on the Success View, is not a single success or a single failure. Rather, it is the *proportion* of successes among all attempts. If the types of possible failures just mentioned are exceptional, then Jaster's Success View can deal with them. If they were exceptional, then they would not count for much in a sufficiently large set of attempts. However, it seems that only (2) and (3) are exceptional failures. Not putting enough effort into trying to φ is not an exception. Instead, it is precisely something that we want to distinguish from lacking the ability to φ. Quite often, we ask ourselves whether we "truly" cannot φ or whether we simply did not try hard enough. Because of this, I suggest that we restrict the relevant possible situations to those in which S *sincerely* tries to φ. That is, S intends to φ and puts sufficient effort into initiating and exercising φ. What counts as "sufficient" will be determined by context and is dependent on normative considerations regarding the effort we expect individuals to put into their attempt to φ.

It is worth emphasizing that S's ability to φ is determined by what S does and would do in a range of relevant possible situations. The fact that an individual has a good track record of φ-ing provides us with a reason to believe that they, in fact, have the ability to φ. That said, we should be cautious when judging individuals' abilities. This is because the fact that S does not φ does not necessarily give us a reason to believe that S lacks the ability to φ. There are different possible explanations when an individual does not φ. One needs to ask "did S put the expected effort in trying to φ?", "did S make some inadvertent mistake?", or "did some accident come between S's initiating the action and the action's completion?" Any assessment of mental disorder cases will have to take such alternative explanations into account.

Thus far, I have mainly discussed agentive abilities. However, as mentioned, not all mental disorders are disorders of action. Many affect our abilities to form (or not form) certain attitudes (for example, beliefs, desires, or emotions). These are not agentive abilities. In these cases, we can apply a version of Jaster's (2020, 160) view on non-agentive abilities:

SUCCESS$_{NAA}$ S has a non-agentive ability to be engaged in some behavior φ if and only if S φs in a sufficiently high proportion of the relevant possible situations in which some S-trigger for φ-ing is present (where the set of the relevant possible situations will vary across ascriber contexts).

To clarify, an "S-trigger is a trigger for φ-ing, in response to which φ-ing is a success" (Jaster 2020, 154). For illustration, consider the ability to digest food. This is a (non-agentive) ability because digesting food counts as a success in response to ingesting food. Why does this count as a success? Because, arguably, it is the biological function of an individual's digestive system to digest food.

Now, what are the relevant success conditions for forming certain attitudes? Regarding actions, Jaster refers to an individual's intentions: "actions are successful insofar as they realize an individual's intentions" (2020, 160). But what are the relevant S-triggers for attitudes? When does forming a certain attitude count as a success? Jaster does not tell us. Here, though, is a proposal. The relevant S-triggers for attitudes are an individual's available (apparent) reasons for or against the attitude in question. I argue for this view in Section 4.5. There, I explicate the sense in which an individual's fear in an anxiety disorder is "excessive." Before doing so, let me discuss the concepts of REASONS and HARM.

4.3 Reasons

The second basic idea behind RHA is that mental disorder involves φ-ings that are sensitive to reasons. For some φ-ing to be "sensitive to reasons" means that it makes sense to ask a certain question "why?" with respect to that φ-ing (see Anscombe 1957, 9). There are, at least, three different types of why-questions, but only two reveal the requisite "sensitivity to reasons." Compare the following examples:

1 *Evidential Reasons*: "The last train to Berlin leaves before midnight." "Why should I believe that?" "That's what the schedule says."
2 *Reasons for Action*: "Jen is considering buying a gift for Berislav." "Why would she do that?" "To cheer him up."
3 *Mere Causes*: "The candle went out." "Why did that happen?" "There was a draft."

Answers to the types of questions asked in (1) and (2) are typically called "normative" or "justifying" reasons. The answer in (3) is only superficially similar to (1) and (2). A why question—as in (1) or (2)—can only be meaningfully asked for attitudes and actions. It is only for attitudes and actions that normative reasons can be meaningfully asked for and offered. Mere events or processes, like a candle going out, can be explained by referring to causes, but it does not make sense to ask for or offer normative reasons for or against them. Thus, it would be misleading to call the things we refer to in (3) "reasons," even if (3) involves an answer to a type of why question. To avoid misunderstandings, it is then better to call them "mere causes."

The prevailing view of normative reasons—as in (1) and (2)—is the following:

REASON   A fact (or alternatively, a true proposition) gives us a normative reason when it *counts in favor* of (or against) our responding in some way, where the response is an attitude (of some type) or an action (of some type).[21]

Thus, normative reasons support a response (of some type). Normative reasons are *pro tanto* reasons. A *pro tanto* reason for a response A can be outweighed by a *pro tanto* reason against response A. If S has *sufficient reason* for a response (of some type), then S is justified in exhibiting that response. If S has *decisive reason* (or most reason) for a response (of some type), then S should exhibit that response (see Kiesewetter 2017, 8-9). A given response can be "adequate" or "inadequate" in the sense that it corresponds or does not correspond to the type of response which one's normative reasons support.

Actions are rationally evaluable with respect to the practical normative reasons we have for them. In other words, an action is rationally evaluable with respect to the facts (or true proposition) that count in favor of that action being worthy of pursuit. S can deliberate on the *pro tanto* reasons they have for or against some action φ. S can weigh these reasons against one another and settle the question of whether, all things considered, they have sufficient (or decisive) reason to φ. Attitudes (like beliefs or emotions) are rationally evaluable with respect to (1) whether they "fit together" (that is, whether they are consistent or coherent with one another) and (2) the situation one is in (that is, with respect to the facts that count in favor of the belief being true or the emotion being objectively adequate).

On the prevailing view, a fact gives us a normative reason when it counts in favor of our responding in some way, regardless of whether we have a belief related to that fact. But the normative reasons an individual has must be present or at least in some sense "available" (Kiesewetter 2017, 161) to them (as, say, dispositions in memory) for those reasons to play a role in the individual's reasoning or deliberating about what to do or what to believe. The fact that I have a nut allergy gives me a normative reason not to eat nuts, regardless of whether I am aware of that fact (see Parfit 2011, 17). Indeed, I need not even believe that I have such an allergy. That said, I cannot (be expected to) respond to the normative reason that the relevant fact gives me if I do not believe that I have a nut allergy (or have that reason in some sense "available" to me). This is why the relevant abilities in mental disorder are abilities to respond adequately to one's *available* reasons. Having knowledge of a normative reason is sufficient for it to be available to the knower.

Why should we believe that normative reasons are given by facts (or true propositions)? The answer is that false propositions cannot count in favor of anything.[22] Consider Derek Parfit's example:

> Suppose that, while walking in some desert, you have disturbed and angered a poisonous snake. You believe that, to save your life, you must run away. In fact, you must stand still, since this snake will attack only moving targets.

(2011, 70)

Do you have a reason to run away? In some sense of "reason," your false belief that running away would save your life gives you a reason—a motivating reason—to run away. A motivating reason is the reason *for which* you run away. And, it is (in part) given by a belief that you take to be true and to count in favor of running away. Your running away is then "rational" (in the instrumental sense). However, as Parfit argues, your motivating reason is one without normative force because it does not count in favor of your response. Reasons that have no normative force should not count as normative reasons. Parfit concludes that false beliefs can, at best, give us *apparent (normative) reasons*. An apparent reason is given by a proposition that would count in favor of responding a certain way if it were true.[23]

A word on "motivating" and "explanatory" reasons (for action).[24] In contrast to normative reasons, motivating reasons need not count in favor of an action. Suppose that you did run away in Parfit's example. What do we need to explain your action in terms of reasons? According to Donald Davidson (1963), motivating reasons are pairs of beliefs and desires. We can explain your action of running away by referring to (1) your desire (or, more generally, your pro-attitude) to save your life and (2) your belief that running away will save your life. Taken together, your desire and belief explain your action by "rationalizing" it, in the sense that they render your running away instrumentally coherent for fulfilling your desire. For Davidson, it is sufficient to show that the response was instrumentally coherent in light of the individual's beliefs and desires to explain an action in terms of reasons. Whether the beliefs and desires count in favor of the response being good or worthy of pursuit is a separate issue.

How do motivating and normative reasons relate to each other? Is there a common core meaning of "reason"? Answering this question is a highly complex undertaking. Nonetheless, I propose the following view. Roughly, a reason is given to us by a proposition playing a certain counting-in-favor-of-φ-ing role. Such a proposition might be one of the following:

1 *Motivating Reason*: A proposition p that S takes to be true and to count in favor of φ-ing, and for which S φs.
2 *Apparent Normative Reason*: A proposition p that S takes to be true and that, if true, would count in favor of S φ-ing.
3 *Normative Reason*: A proposition p that is true and counts in favor of S φ-ing.

On this view, an individual S might have a motivating reason where the proposition p gives them either an apparent normative reason or a normative reason (or neither of these). There are also no reasons *tout court*. When we ask "did S have a reason to φ?", we must specify the sense of "reason" we are interested in.

On RHA, it is the normative and apparent normative reasons that are relevant. Nevertheless, we should keep in mind that (1) explaining an individual's actions in light of their motivating reasons and (2) evaluating their actions in light of their normative reasons are two different projects. RHA does not imply that we cannot explain (or even rationalize) the attitudes and actions of individuals with mental disorder in light of their motivating reasons. Individuals with mental disorders may have attitudes and perform actions that are to a large extent rational from their point of view. But something is awry with the relationship between (a) their attitudes or actions and (b) their (available) normative or apparent normative reasons.

There is a potential worry with the claim that the φ-ings involved in mental disorder are those that are sensitive to reasons. A skeptic might object that this claim yields some obviously false verdicts. It might entail, for instance, that mood disorders are not mental disorders. This is because, on the prevailing view, moods such as depressiveness are not sensitive to reasons. Moods are often distinguished from emotions, and it is relatively uncontroversial that emotions (for example, sadness) are sensitive to reasons (in the aforementioned sense). However, it is controversial whether moods are. Emotions can be objectively adequate or inadequate (see Section 4.5), and they can "fit" or "not fit" our beliefs. However, things appear to be different when it comes to moods. When you wake up in a good mood, you need not think that you have a reason for being in a good mood. You might just happen to be in a good mood. In this case, your mood does not seem to be *about* anything. *Prima facie*, RHA maintains that mood disorders are not mental disorders.

But, this line of thinking involves an implausible view of many moods. I argue that moods like depressiveness are generally sensitive to reasons. This is because, generally, it makes sense to ask an individual for their reasons for or against being in a particular mood. The mere fact that we often do not think about or know why we are in a particular mood does not mean that the question does not apply. Perhaps, the question does not apply to certain moods (like waking up in a good mood). But, as Jesse Prinz (2004) argues, moods can be objectively adequate or inadequate in light of how life is going for the affected individual quite generally. Prinz argues that the difference between emotions and moods is not whether they represent (or whether they are intentional states). It is rather *what* they represent: "Sadness represents a particular loss, while depression represents a losing battle" (Prinz 2004, 185).

4.4 Harm

According to RHA, having a mental disorder necessarily involves harm. (Recall that my aim is to explicate the concept MENTAL DISORDER for scientific and normative purposes, see Section 1.2.) I contrast "harm" with living a "good life" or a "life worth living."[25] I use these expressions as overarching terms for all things that make an individual's life a non-instrumentally good one or a life worth living *for the individual who lives it.*[26] What does it mean to be "harmed" and what kinds of things are harms? Before discussing these questions, let me briefly introduce some terminology and some distinctions.

An event *e* (or a property of *e* or a continuant participating in *e*) that causes an individual S harm in some respect X (where X is a component of what makes S's life a non-instrumentally good one for S) is a "harmful event."[27] An individual S who is caused some harm in some respect X by some event *e* is "harmed." For example, a car crash causes S to have a painful fracture. This is a harm to S in some respect because it is painful. We can say that the car crash is a "harmful event," that S was "harmed," and that the painful injury is a "harm." Furthermore, I take it that, if S is in a bad state, S is "harmed," in the sense that S is subject to harm. Since harm comes in degrees, I understand the locution "to be harmed" as "to be harmed to a sufficient degree." Different dimensions seem to be involved. Pain can vary in both intensity and duration; both these dimensions appear relevant for assessing a pain's severity.

Some event (or state) can either be *instrumentally* or *non-instrumentally* good or bad for an individual.[28] An event is non-instrumentally good for an individual if it has value for them *in itself.* An event is instrumentally good if it has value for an individual *for the sake of something else.*[29] For example, dancing is non-instrumentally good for an individual if it has value for them in itself. Having a fever can be instrumentally good for an individual if it has value for them for the sake of something else, say, to avoid a difficult meeting at work. Something can, at the same time, be non-instrumentally harmful and instrumentally beneficial to an individual. Imagine someone who vomits after swallowing poison. Because vomiting is uncomfortable, it is non-instrumentally harmful. But, because vomiting prevents further discomfort (from the poison), it is, at the same time, instrumentally beneficial.

Harm and beneficence are not exhaustive. Some events may be neither harmful nor beneficial to an individual. That I am working on my book today is neither harmful nor beneficial to LeBron James in any respect whatsoever. Moreover, harm should also be distinguished from a mere deprivation of good. An individual deprived of a good is not necessarily harmed. An individual who does not win the lottery is deprived of a good, but they are not obviously harmed in any respect. However, it is possible that an individual who is prevented from receiving a good is harmed (for example, when it leaves them in a state that was bad to begin with). Matthew Hanser offers the following example:

Suppose that a doctor fails to perform an operation that would have restored a blind person's sight. Had the doctor not failed to perform the operation—that is, had he performed it—the patient would have been better off in an important respect.

(2008, 427)

An individual can be *pro tanto* or *all things considered* harmed by an event. A visit to a dentist can be *pro tanto* harmful because it typically involves unpleasant or painful experiences. But the same visit can be *pro tanto* harmless or even beneficent because it ultimately prevents further unpleasant or painful experiences related to tooth decay (Bradley 2012, 393).[30] Events can also be harmless (or harmful) in the short-term, but harmful (or harmless) in the long-term. Smoking one cigarette probably never killed anyone, but smoking cigarettes on a regular basis is harmful for smokers in the long-term.

It is plausible that an individual's mental disorder can be instrumentally beneficent to them (for example, they might be more creative). Also, they need not be harmed by their condition, all things considered (recall the happy philosopher with an anxiety disorder from Chapter 2). Nonetheless, I hold that, for a condition to fall under MENTAL DISORDER, it must be (instrumentally or non-instrumentally) harmful to S in some relevant respect.

What does it mean to be "harmed"? There are three prominent views:

1 *Non-Comparative Accounts (NCA)*: An individual is harmed if and only if they are in a non-comparatively bad state.[31]
2 *Counterfactual Comparative Accounts (CCA)*: An individual is harmed by an event *e* if and only if they are worse off in some respect than they would have been if *e* had not occurred.
3 *Temporal Comparative Accounts (TCA)*: An individual is harmed by an event *e* if and only if they are worse off in some respect than they were before *e* occurred.[32]

All three proposals face certain counterexamples. NCAs have trouble capturing cases in which an individual is harmed by an event (say, a stroke) that does not leave them in a non-comparatively bad state (say, with decreased but still average intellectual abilities, see Thomson 2011, 439). CCAs have well-known troubles with (1) cases of overdetermination (two events simultaneously cause a certain effect, each of them being sufficient for the effect to occur) and (2) preemption (see Parfit 1984, chapter 3, Hanser 2008, Bradley 2012, Klocksiem 2012, and Feit 2015). Both CCAs and TCAs have trouble with genetic diseases, where an individual would not have existed without the disease (see Parfit 1984, chapter 16 and Boorse 2011, 52).

Here, I do not settle on any of these accounts. This is because (1), as far as I can tell, we cannot yet make a final judgment regarding which account is correct and (2), in principle, RHA is not committed to any particular account of what it means to be "harmed." I shall therefore merely note some sufficient conditions for being harmed. The consequence is that we might miss some cases of harm and thus get some false negative verdicts on the presence of a mental disorder. Nonetheless, the sufficient conditions I will mention surely capture a large number of the phenomena that fall under MENTAL DISORDER.

I propose that for an individual S to be harmed by their condition C in some respect X it is sufficient that

i C is non-instrumentally bad for S in some respect X;
ii C causes S to be sufficiently worse off than before or than S would have otherwise been in respect X; or
iii C prevents S from receiving a good in respect X and thereby leaves S in a non-instrumentally bad state in respect X, *where X is some component of what makes S's life a non-instrumentally good one for S.*

A comprehensive view of mental disorder will have to be supplemented by a substantive theory about (1) what makes an individual's life a non-instrumentally good one and (2) which of these components are relevant in the psychiatric and psychotherapeutic context. The fact that different authors in the philosophy of medicine and psychiatry offer different lists of harms indicates that this is a difficult task. For example, Gert, Culver, and Clouser (2006, 142 f.) put death, pain, disability (or loss of ability), loss of freedom, and loss of pleasure on their list. The *DSM-5* lists distress (or suffering) and "disability in social, occupational, or other important activities" (APA 2013, 20). Nordenfelt (1995, 60 ff., 75) introduces the idea of "minimal human happiness," which includes the needs humans share with other living beings (for example, the need for food, having a sheltered home, some economic security, some intellectual pleasures, and some pleasures of bodily locomotion), but excludes an individual's self-chosen goals (for example, becoming a professional dancer or philosophy professor).

In principle, RHA is not committed to any particular substantive theory of living a good life. Providing such a theory also exceeds the scope of this book. It would though be disappointing to leave the question of what it is for an individual to live a good life entirely open. I shall therefore give some thoughts on the issue. I do so by way of discussing subjectivist, objectivist, and hybrid views.

According to subjectivist views (desire-fulfillment theories and preference-hedonism), the standard for evaluating how well an individual's life is going for them is their desires and only their desires.[33] According to objectivist views, the standard is *not* an individual's desires. Rather, "certain things are good or bad for people, whether or not these people would want to have the good things, or to avoid the bad things" (Parfit 1984, 499). According to hybrid views, the standard for evaluating how well an individual's life is going for them is a composite of (1) wanting (2) good things (and wanting to avoid bad things). In the following, I argue for the hybrid view, although I cannot provide a full defense here.

Parfit (1984) argues that we should prefer *global* versions of desire-fulfillment theories or preference-hedonism over *summative* ones. The former appeal only to an individual's desires about some part of their life (considered as a whole) or about their whole life. Parfit gives the following example to argue for this view:

> Suppose that I could either have fifty years of life of an extremely high quality, or an indefinite number of years that are barely worth living. In the first alternative, my fifty years would, on any theory, go extremely well. I would be very happy, would achieve great things, do much good, and love and be loved by many people. In the second alternative my life would always be, though not by much, worth living. There would be nothing bad about this life, and it would each day contain a few small pleasures.
>
> (1984, 498)

On the summative version of desire-fulfillment theories or preference-hedonism, the second alternative only needs to be long enough to make it a better life than the first one. But this, Parfit holds, is implausible. On the global version of subjectivism, what makes S's life go best depends on what S would prefer, now and in the various alternatives if S knew all relevant facts about these alternatives.

A problem for subjectivist views is that they yield unacceptable claims about cases in which S has fully informed desires to devote their life to pursuing trivial ends (for example, counting blades of grass, see Rawls 1971, 432) or immoral ends (for example, causing others pain without consent). Subjectivist views imply that S is faring well when pursuing such ends, but it does not seem that they are. However, this argument is inconclusive because the subjectivist might respond that it simply begs the question.

Another problem for subjectivist views is that they cannot justify certain normative consequences of being harmed. If harm justifies, in part, (1) why an individual with a mental disorder has a *pro tanto* reason to seek treatment and (2) why other people have a *pro tanto* reason to treat them with greater care, then being harmed cannot amount to a lack of desire fulfillment. This is because not all desires make demands on other individuals. As James Griffin puts it, "mere desires are morally lightweight" (1986, 46).

Furthermore, if desires do not provide normative reasons, then "it is odd to claim that the factors that make something contribute to one's well-being do not provide reasons for pursuing it" (Scanlon 1998, 114).

However, objectivist views are also problematic. A problem for objectivist views is that they overlook the importance of an individual's experiences, and they fail to respect individual preferences and autonomy (see Railton 2003, 47). Objective goods may be important, but they do not necessarily lead to a good life for the individual who lives it if they do not correspond to the experiences or preferences of the individual living that life. Consider having knowledge or engaging in rational activity:

> 'Would these states of mind be good, if they brought no enjoyment, and if the person in these states of mind had not the slightest desire that they continue?' The answer is no.
>
> (Parfit 1984, 501)

Simply put, if an individual does not want "more of this!" given the life they live, then it does not seem to be a good life *for them*.

Another problem for objectivist views is that they have difficulties determining what constitutes objective goods or values. Wolf points out that there is a danger of elitism

> *Who's to say* which projects are fitting (or worthy or valuable) and which are not? The worry is that the views of any one person or any group that sets itself up as an authority on values are liable to be narrow-minded or biased.
>
> (2010, 39)

So, there is a danger of thinking that one knows which things are objectively good or valuable when one is, in fact, simply expressing one's subjective views.

Hybrid views avoid the problems mentioned for subjectivist views and the first of the problems mentioned for objectivist views. This is why I am inclined toward a hybrid view. However, they still face the second problem mentioned for objectivist views. Wolf, who defends a hybrid view about *meaningfulness*, concedes that there is simply no final authority about which things have value. But, on Wolf's view,

> the absence of a final authority [...] does not call into doubt the legitimacy or coherence of the question itself or the enterprise of trying to find a more or less reasonable, if also partial, tentative, and impermanent answer.
>
> (2010, 40)

So, what should a proponent of a hybrid theory do? According to Wolf, the questions "are open to anyone to ask and to try to answer" (2010, 39). We should basically engage in a potentially never-ending enterprise of giving reasons for why certain things are valuable to us. This conclusion might be disappointing. But I think that it accurately reflects the fact that there simply is no easy answer to the question of what makes an individual's life a non-instrumentally good one.

To end this section, let me point out three harms that seem particularly relevant in the context of psychiatry and psychotherapy: (1) pain and suffering, (2) lack of autonomy, and (3) lack of meaningfulness.

Pain and Suffering. On all plausible substantive theories, a component that makes S's life non-instrumentally good is being happy and avoiding pain and suffering. Suffering comes in various forms. These include:

- panic/fear, distress, or pain (torture, threats)
- sadness or grief (lovesickness, death of a loved one)
- anxiety (job loss, financial insecurity, loss of one's home)
- loneliness (absence or loss of friends or family)
- guilt (betrayal)
- shame (failure to achieve a self-determined goal)
- regret (not having children)
- resentfulness (toward a neglectful parent)
- reluctance (being in a situation that one does not want to be in, such as having an unwanted child)
- jealousy (a loved one is having an affair)

At a minimum, to suffer is to have a negatively valenced ("less of this!") feeling (sensation, mood, or emotion). Suffering does not necessarily come with high arousal. It is possible to suffer because one is bored to death.

One specific way in which we can suffer is when we have frustrated desires. On a semantic view of what it is for a desire to be "satisfied," my desire to eat chocolate is satisfied when I eat chocolate, and it is not satisfied when I do not. We must distinguish this sense of being "satisfied"—or better "fulfilled"—from experiencing a feeling of satisfaction. It is possible for desire fulfillment and satisfaction to come apart. It is possible to have a desire fulfilled but not feel satisfied by it. Conversely, it is possible to have an unfulfilled desire but be satisfied anyway (I may find a substitute or not care too much about the desire).

Lack of Autonomy. Consider a situation in which S cannot do what they want to do because of their mental constitution, and S cannot come to terms with their inability. Let us say that S cannot stop picking their skin, although they desperately want to. They cannot get rid of their desire and they cannot stop feeling frustrated about the fact that they cannot.

Furthermore, they feel hopeless that they might get rid of the mental constitution that causes them to pick their skin. This seems like a typical pattern in mental disorder. Such a condition is bad for the individual because (1) they suffer, and (2) it impairs their autonomy (in the sense that it impairs their ability to think and decide for themselves what to do and how to live). On the assumption that autonomy is a component of (or a precondition for) what makes an individual's life a non-instrumentally good one, an individual is harmed (in a mental disorder–relevant sense) when they suffer and their condition impairs their autonomy to a sufficient degree.

Lack of Meaningfulness. Individuals can be harmed in a mental disorder–relevant sense when their condition impairs their ability to achieve meaningfulness in their life. According to Wolf, "meaning arises from loving objects worthy of love and engaging with them in a positive way" (2010, 8). Wolf identifies three requirements for meaningfulness: (1) the subject must love (be gripped, excited by) the object, (2) the object must be worthy of love, and (3) the subject must relate actively to the object, that is, not just recognize it, but "create it, protect it, promote it, honor it, or more generally [...] actively affirm it in some way or other" (2010, 10). Being able to actively engage with an object worthy of love is highly demanding in the sense that it requires a lot of mental resources (attention, forming intentions, planning, etc.). Individuals with mental disorder often lack such resources.

4.5 Case Study: Anxiety Disorder

In Section 4.3, I suggested that the relevant success conditions for attitudes (for example, beliefs and emotions) are an individual's available (apparent) reasons. I now flesh out this claim by way of an example. Consider Fiona, an individual suffering from panic disorder with agoraphobia (a type of anxiety disorder). Fiona often experiences high-intensity fear of dying. During these episodes, she experiences increased heartrate, vertigo, dizziness, heavy trembling, and profuse sweating. She mostly experiences these fears when she is at home alone or when she leaves her home. Fiona also avoids almost all public spaces, such as supermarkets, shopping streets, and public transportation. She leaves the house only in the company of her husband and/or daughter. Something about Fiona's fear is clearly "disordered." The *DSM-5* spells this out in terms of "excessiveness." Anxiety disorders are mainly characterized by "excessive fear and anxiety and related behavioral disturbances" (APA 2013, 189).[34] But, in what sense is Fiona's fear "excessive," and how does this relate to RHA?

Let me first make some general remarks on fear. Fear is an emotion that typically alerts us to and motivates us to flee from danger (see Lazarus 1991, 1999).[35] When I experience fear, my fear represents some situation as dangerous for me. When I am confronted by a teeth-fletching and snarling dog, my fear represents that situation (the dog fletching its teeth and snarling) as dangerous for me. The degree of intensity of my fear represents the degree of perceived danger. A highly intense fear represents a situation as highly dangerous, while a minimally intense fear represents a situation as minimally dangerous.

Fear can be objectively adequate or inadequate. My fear is objectively inadequate when it "misrepresents" a situation, that is, when the situation is, in fact, not dangerous. My fear is also (partly) objectively inadequate when I experience a high degree of fear in a situation that is, in fact, only slightly dangerous.

Given the aforementioned, one might propose the following view of anxiety disorder:

ANXIETY$_{\text{INADEQUACY}}$ An individual S has an anxiety disorder only if

    i   S experiences fear with sufficient frequency in situations $c_1, c_2, ..., c_n$ and

    ii   S's fear in situations $c_1, c_2, ..., c_n$ is (at least, partly) objectively inadequate given the degree to which situations $c_1, c_2, ..., c_n$ are, in fact, dangerous for S.

This view fits the *DSM-5* characterization of anxiety disorder: a fear is "excessive" when it is "out of proportion to the actual threat" (APA 2013, 203). On this view, Fiona has an anxiety disorder because she frequently experiences (highly intense) fear in situations in which she is not (or is only minimally) in danger.

Why "sufficient frequency" in (i)? This is because we all misrepresent situations from time to time. Fiona does not have anxiety disorder if she only experiences high-intensity fear in *one* situation in which she is minimally in danger. The more frequently she exhibits such misrepresentations, the more likely it is that she has an anxiety disorder. Thus, anxiety disorder involves more than merely being mistaken in one's fear from time to time. At a minimum, an individual must be mistaken in their fears with sufficient frequency.

Although this might be true of many actual cases, experiencing objectively inadequate fears is neither necessary nor sufficient for having an anxiety disorder. It is not necessary because it is conceptually possible for an individual to have an anxiety disorder and for their fears to be objectively adequate, for example, in cases in which they are in danger but do *not know* or *justifiably believe* it. One can easily imagine cases in which Fiona suddenly experiences intense fear and truly believes that she is in danger but has no available (apparent) reason to believe that she is in danger. In such cases, Fiona's fears would be objectively adequate but still pathological. This is because her fears are inadequate *in light of her epistemic situation.*

Experiencing objectively inadequate fears is also not sufficient for having an anxiety disorder. This is because it is possible for an individual not to have an anxiety disorder even though their fears are objectively inadequate. One can easily imagine cases in which Fiona has every available (apparent) reason to believe that she is in danger even though she is not. There could, after all, be *misleading evidence.* Suppose that Fiona sees a realistic tiger mock-up. This causes her to believe that there is a tiger. Because she also believes that tigers are dangerous, her fear would be subjectively rational. Fiona's belief that there is a tiger gives her sufficient (apparent) reason for her fear. Nevertheless, her fear is objectively inadequate. This is because she is, in fact, not in danger. In such cases, Fiona's fear would not be pathological because her fear is adequate given her epistemic situation.

Because objective inadequacy is neither necessary nor sufficient for having an anxiety disorder, it would be extensionally inadequate to define ANXIETY DISORDER in terms of objective inadequacy. Some clear cases of anxiety disorder would not be captured by the definition, while some clear cases of non-pathological fear would be. Nevertheless, the discussion is not fruitless. It helps us recognize what is crucial for defining ANXIETY DISORDER. It seems that an individual's fears must, in some sense, be "inadequate in light of their epistemic situation" for them to have an anxiety disorder. But, in what sense exactly?

One way to flesh out this thought would be in terms of *consistency* (or *coherence*). One might suggest that what demarcates pathological from non-pathological fear is whether an individual's fears are consistent (or inconsistent) with their beliefs. On this view, anxiety disorder concerns how an individual's attitudes relate to one another and not how they relate to the facts (or states of affairs) they are about. It is the logical-semantic relations among an individual's attitudes that are "disordered."

In light of this, one might propose the following view of anxiety disorder:

ANXIETY$_{\text{INCONSISTENCY}}$ An individual S has an anxiety disorder only if

    i   S experiences fear in situations c_1, c_2, ..., c_n with sufficient frequency and

    ii   S's fear in situations c_1, c_2, ..., c_n is inconsistent with S's beliefs in situations c_1, c_2, ..., c_n.

On this view, Fiona has an anxiety disorder because she frequently experiences fear of dying in situations in which she does not believe that she is in danger. As such, she appears to have inconsistent mental attitudes. By experiencing fear in a certain situation, Fiona represents that situation as being dangerous. By believing (in the same situation) that she is not in danger, Fiona represents that situation as not being dangerous. Representing a situation (via an emotion) as dangerous to oneself *and* representing that same situation (via a belief) as not dangerous to oneself is irrational, because that a situation is at the same time (dangerous and not dangerous to oneself) is inconsistent. On such an account, having a pathological mental condition would amount to something like being subject to frequent instances of obvious (partial) inconsistency.

Although inconsistency of this sort is often *de facto* involved in anxiety disorder, it is not necessary for having it. At least, *obvious* (partial) inconsistency is not necessary. This is because it is possible for an individual to have an anxiety disorder and to have a *prima facie* consistent set of beliefs. Imagine that Fiona frequently experiences fear when sitting in a quiet library. She believes that she is in danger and that she has sufficient reason for this belief. In other words, not only does she have the belief that she is in danger, but she also has other beliefs that she takes to constitute sufficient reason for that belief. In this case, Fiona's fears and beliefs form a, *prima facie*, highly consistent set of beliefs. Nevertheless, Fiona might still have an anxiety disorder. But, under which conditions? I propose the following: an individual has an anxiety disorder only if they do not respond to their available (apparent) reasons in a suitable way; that is, if they do not respond to those of their beliefs that give them available (apparent) reasons against their fear (when those beliefs are, in fact, giving them such reasons).

In Section 4.3, I stated that an apparent reason is a proposition that would count in favor of our responding in some way if it were true. The belief that there is a poisonous snake in front of you gives you an apparent reason to experience fear. This is because the proposition expressed in that belief (if true) counts in favor of your responding with fear. Poisonous snakes are, after all, dangerous to us. By contrast, the belief that there are trees in the woods does not give you an apparent reason to experience fear.

There are, then, two ways in which an individual can fail to respond adequately to their available (apparent) reasons:

1 by responding to a belief as giving them a reason when it actually does *not* (not even an apparent one) or
2 by *not* responding to a belief as giving them a reason when it actually does (at least, an apparent one).

Consider an individual who believes that there is a sofa and thinks that this gives them a reason for their belief that there will be a World War III. Even if their belief that there is a sofa is true, it does not support their belief that there will be a World War III. This is because the propositions expressed in these beliefs do not stand in any justification-relevant relationship to each other. The individual responds to some belief as giving them a reason but it actually does not give them a reason (not even an apparent one).

By contrast, consider an individual who believes that something is, in a medical sense, "not okay" with their heart. After a medical examination, their cardiologist tells them that their heart is fine. Imagine that the individual then simply ignores the cardiologist's evaluation. Perhaps, they think "well, why should a doctor know better than me?" In this case, the individual does not think that their one belief—that the cardiologist judged their heart to be fine—gives them a reason against their other belief—that something is "not OK" with their heart. But actually, it does give them such a reason (at least an apparent one).[36]

Let me return to the case of Fiona. In what sense is Fiona's fear inadequate in light of her epistemic situation? It cannot be that Fiona does not have sufficient reason for her fear. That an individual does not have sufficient reason for their fear is not necessary for having an anxiety disorder. It is possible that they do not have sufficient reason for their fear but their fear is not pathological. Recall that Fiona sees a realistic tiger mock-up and believes that there is a real tiger. Given her belief that there is a tiger, Fiona comes to believe that she is in danger. As a consequence, she also experiences fear. In this case, Fiona does not have sufficient reason for her fear, because her belief that there is a tiger does not give her a reason to begin with (it gives her only an apparent reason). Her belief is false, and false beliefs do not support anything. Nevertheless, Fiona's fear is not pathological because there is nothing intrinsically "not OK" with her. Fiona's reasoning is fine; it is just that the "input" (the initial belief) is false. Even more, Fiona has good apparent reason for her fear. Her belief that there is a tiger would support her belief that she is in danger if the former were true. So, her fear is perfectly adequate in light of her epistemic situation. In other words, her fear—although objectively inadequate and not sufficiently supported by reasons—is subjectively rational. And this suffices to make it non-pathological.

Now, imagine that Fiona does not even have an apparent reason for her fear. That is, imagine that she responds to some of her beliefs as giving her a reason for her fear when, in fact, they do not. This is not because the beliefs are false, but because they do not stand in the counting-in-favor relation. Imagine that Fiona believes that she is in danger because there are trees in the woods. Again, her belief that there are trees in the woods is true, but it does not support her fear. That there are trees in the woods does not count in favor of her belief that she is in danger. These propositions simply do not stand in a justification-relevant relationship to each other. In this case, Fiona's fears are pathological because they are inadequate in light of her epistemic situation (there is not even an apparent reason for her fear).

Although Fiona's fears surely seem pathological, it is not so clear whether her fears indicate an anxiety disorder. One might think that such cases exemplify something like a delusion. Perhaps, cases in which an individual responds to some of their beliefs as giving them reasons for their fear when they do not are not typical of anxiety disorder. A typical case would be the following. Fiona consults a cardiologist who tells her that her heart is fine. Fiona comes to believe that her doctor told her that her heart is fine but does not respond to this belief as giving her (a) a reason against her belief that she is in danger or (b) a reason against her fear. That is, Fiona keeps on believing that she is in danger or experiencing fear.

In light of this, one might propose the following view of anxiety disorder:

ANXIET$_{\text{RESPONSE}}$ An individual S has an anxiety disorder only if

> i   S experiences fear in situations $c_1, c_2, ..., c_n$ with sufficient frequency;
>
> ii S has beliefs that give them sufficient (apparent) reason against their fear in situations $c_1, c_2, ..., c_n$; and
>
> iii S does not respond to those beliefs that *de facto* give them sufficient (apparent) reason against their fear in situations $c_1, c_2, ..., c_n$ as giving them sufficient reasons against their fear in situations $c_1, c_2, ..., c_n$.

However, the fact that an individual does not *take* those beliefs that give them sufficient (apparent) reason against their fear to *be* such reasons against their fear does not guarantee that they have an anxiety disorder. They may simply have a "bad track record" when it comes to responding adequately to their available (apparent) reasons without anything being intrinsically "not OK" or "disordered." I contend that invoking the notion of ability provides the best way to understand the difference between these two types of cases: simply having a "bad track record" versus having a disorder.

More specifically, I propose the following view of anxiety disorder:

ANXIETY$_{\text{RHA}}$ An individual S has an anxiety disorder if and only if

> i   S experiences fear in situations $c_1, c_2, ..., c_n$ with sufficient frequency;
>
> ii S has beliefs that give them sufficient (apparent) reason against their fear in situations $c_1, c_2, ..., c_n$;

    iii   S lacks the ability not to experience fear in situations in which S has beliefs that give them sufficient (apparent) reason against their fear in situations $c_1, c_2, ..., c_n$; and

    iv   S is harmed by their condition.

On RHA, Fiona has an anxiety disorder if and only if (1) she lacks the ability to respond adequately to her available (apparent) reasons for (or against) her fear in view of her mental constitution and her life circumstances, and (2) she is harmed by her condition.

How does RHA's account of anxiety disorder differ from the *DSM-5* characterization? And, why is the former preferable to the latter? As already mentioned, the view behind the *DSM-5* characterization of anxiety disorder seems to be ANXIETY$_{\text{INADEQUACY}}$. On this view, excessiveness is measured against what is objectively adequate, that is, with respect to the actual threat. By contrast, on RHA, excessiveness is measured against the individual's epistemic situation. On this view, we need to evaluate whether an individual's mental attitudes make sense in light of their epistemic situation to determine whether they have an anxiety disorder. RHA is preferable to ANXIETY$_{\text{INADEQUACY}}$, because it does not fall prey to the same counterexamples.

4.6 The Full View

Here is a more detailed version of RHA for the clearest (types of) cases that should fall under MENTAL DISORDER (see Section 5.2 for an expansion of RHA to other cases):

RHA$_{\text{PSY}}$ An individual S has a mental disorder if and only if

    i   S does not have the ability to respond adequately to some of their available (apparent) reasons for (or against) some of their reason-sensitive attitudes or actions; *in view of* their mental constitution and their life circumstances (where the threshold of inability is determined by the degree at which individuals in the relevant comparison class are, on average, harmed by their condition C in some respect X) and

    ii   S is harmed by their condition C in some respect X, *where X is some component of what makes S's life a non-instrumentally good one for S.*

For S to be harmed by C in some respect X it is sufficient that

i C is non-instrumentally bad for S in some respect X;

ii C causes S to be sufficiently worse off than before or than they would otherwise have been in respect X; or iii C prevents S from receiving a good in respect X, thereby leaving S in a non-instrumentally bad state in respect X, *where X is some component of what makes S's life a non-instrumentally good one for S.*

RHA can be spelled out even further with respect to agentive and non-agentive mental disorder.

Here is the full version of RHA for non-agentive mental disorders:

RHA_{NA}   An individual S has a (non-agentive) mental disorder if and only if

    i   S is sufficiently frequently (or continuously) in a manifest reasons-sensitive mental state of type C;

    ii   S has beliefs that give them sufficient available (apparent) reason against C;

    iii   S does not have the (non-agentive) ability to change C, where the relevant possible situations are those in which

        a   S has beliefs that give them sufficient available (apparent) reason against C;

        b   S is in the same mental constitution and life circumstances as in actual situations in which they are in C; and

    iv   S is harmed by their condition C in some respect X, *where X is some component of what makes S's life a non-instrumentally good one for S.*

Here is the full version of RHA for agentive mental disorders:

RHA_A   An individual S has an (agentive) mental disorder if and only if

    i   S φs sufficiently frequently (where φ-ing is an action);

    ii   S does not have the (agentive) ability to omit φ-ing, where the relevant possible situations are those in which

        a   S has beliefs that give them sufficient available (apparent) reasons against φ-ing;

        b   S sincerely tries not to φ;

        c   S is in the same mental constitution and life circumstances as in their actual situation; and

    iii   S is harmed by their condition C in some respect X, *where X is some component of what makes S's life a non-instrumentally good one for S.*

Given the aforementioned, it is relatively easy to see which dimensions are relevant for assessing the severity of a mental disorder. It depends on:

1 the frequency of either manifest mental state C or φ-ing;
2 the degree of ability (where both the modal success rate and the range of contexts is relevant); and
3 the degree of harm (where both the intensity and duration are relevant).

For example, a high frequency of φ-ing, a low degree of ability to omit φ-ing, and a high degree of harm, *ceteris paribus*, suggest that the individual has a rather severe mental disorder.

Notes

1 Parts of this chapter draw on Dembić (2023).
2 I will provide a more general version of RHA, one that also applies to what I call "psychosomatic" and "somatopsychic" disorders, in Section 5.2.
3 See Edwards (1981), Bolton (2001), Gaete (2008), and Graham (2010) for similar views. According to Edwards, mental disorder involves a "prolonged inability to know and deal in a rational and autonomous way with oneself and one's social and physical environment" (1981, 312). According to Bolton, it has to do "with a 'radical failure' of intentionality" (2001, 185). According to Gaete, S has a mental disorder if and only if S "(a) lacks (a certain degree of) some (mental) capacity or capacities that she is expected to possess given her age and her culture, and (b) her lacking in such a capacity (or set of capacities) is causing her some sort of harm" (2008, 331). Graham holds that the "inability or impairment that is distinctive of a mental disorder is that the subject behaves, and cannot but behave, in various *irrational, unreasonable* or *reason-unresponsive* (or *unwarranted* and so on) ways" (2010, 117). See Bortolotti (2013) for a critique of Edwards' (1981) view. See Varga (2017) for a critique of Graham's (2010) view.
4 φ-ings can be actions or non-agentive events or processes. The locution "S does not have the ability to φ" means "S does not have the ability to φ to a sufficient degree." It does *not* necessarily mean "S does not have the ability to φ *at all*" (see Section 4.2).
5 If one believes that "having" certain reasons already entails that those reasons are, in some sense, "available" to the agent, then noting that they are "available" is redundant. I will explain "available" and "apparent" in Section 4.3.
6 Seminal works on generic statements include Leslie (2007, 2008) and Nickel (2016).
7 See Heinz (2014, 333) for a similar point.
8 Barnes (2016) gives this as a counterexample to the idea that a disability equates to an inability.
9 See Gregory (2020) for a similar point with respect to disability.
10 See Arpaly (2005), Gipps (2006), and Graham (2010) for similar points.
11 This overview draws on Jaster (2020, chapter 1).
12 Abilities are characteristically ascribed by using the modal auxiliary "can": "I can run a marathon." But, not all "can"-statements are ascriptions of abilities (Kratzer 1977). In addition to the ability sense of "can," there is also a deontic sense ("you can't kill a cat"), an epistemic sense ("they can't be the murderer"), and many more ("don't go there, you can fall from the roof"). The ability sense of "can" is in play when stating that an individual with a mental disorder "cannot" φ.

13 The concept associated with the term "ability" here is a wide one (see Jaster 2020). Some people might prefer a narrower concept of "ability" that restricts ability ascriptions to actions. On this view, what I have called "non-agentive ability" is better described as "disposition," "capacity," or the like.

14 See Stalnaker (2014) for more on the concept of context.

15 According to Kratzer (1977, 1981), the modal auxiliary "can" is a sentence modifier which modifies a proposition by assigning possibility to it. Usually, "can"-statements express *restricted* possibility. On this view, "S can swim" translates into "It is possible, in a properly restricted sense, that S swims." Spelled out in terms of possible worlds semantics a statement of the form "S can φ" is true if and only if there is at least one possible world, in a properly restricted sense, in which S φs. The phrase "in view of F" is a non-technical way of expressing that the properly restricted possible worlds are those in which the facts F obtain. For a clarification of this point, see also Jaster (2020, 64 f.).

16 Those authors who (1) take sensitivity to reasons to be criterial of agency and (2) claim that emotions are sensitive to reasons would disagree (for example, Moran 2001). However, these writers also typically claim that emotions are not "agentive" in the same sense that an action such as singing is. On their view, the relevant distinction would be the one between (a) voluntary agency and (b) non-voluntary agency and non-agentive processes.

17 See Vihvelin (2013) for a more detailed view of which conditions we typically hold fixed. On her view, the individual has to be "in surroundings where the *extrinsic enablers* (e.g., a bicycle and a place to ride it) for the ability are in place and where there are no *extrinsic masks* (e.g., bicycle bullies lurking in the background) to the exercise of the ability and where the person *retains the intrinsic property B that is the causal basis* of the ability" (2013, 187).

18 See Foucault (1965, 1973, 1977) and Tremain (2015, 2017).

19 It is worth noting that my claim here is not that one can enable an individual with a mental disorder *without* changing their mental constitution, but only that, in principle, changing the individual's mental constitution could also be achieved by changing their external circumstances, see Section 5.1.3.

20 In principle, RHA can be spelled out with any analysis of ABILITY that accounts for the relevant features.

21 See, after Kiesewetter (2017), Scanlon (1998, 17), Dancy (2000, 1), Velleman (2000), Gibbard (2003, 188–89), Finlay (2006, 5), Thomson (2008, 127), Raz (2009, 18), Parfit (2011, 31), and Broome (2013, 54).

22 There is some controversy around whether normative reasons for actions are (a) *attitudes* (that is, beliefs or desires) or (b) propositions, facts, events, or objects that might serve as the *content* of such attitudes (attitudes that the beliefs or desires are about). For a discussion, see Dancy (2000).

23 It is possible that your motivating reason does not even give you an apparent normative reason. Consider the following example: S kills their cat because the cat spilled the milk. Even if this is true, S's cat spilling the milk would not count in favor of S killing the cat. This is because it does not show S's killing the cat to be a worthwhile pursuit.

24 See Dancy (2000) for a discussion of the history of this distinction.

25 "Harm" is often contrasted with "well-being." I choose the expressions "good life" and "life worth living" because there seems to be a concept of "well-being" that is narrower than the one expressed by the former terms. For example, it makes sense to claim that one has sacrificed one's well-being for a life worth living (see Scanlon 1998, 112).

26 Scanlon (1993, 185) contrasts the following two questions: "What makes a life a good one for the person who lives it? What makes a life a valuable one (a good thing, as Sidgwick put it, 'from the point of view of the universe')?" I claim that in the context of mental health and disorder, we care especially about the first question.

27 See Thomson (1997) for the view that whatever is good is good in some respect. A "continuant" in ontology is something that exists and that preserves its identity through time, for example, a car or a person.

28 What is the relation to intrinsic goodness? I follow Zimmerman and Bradley's (2019) suggestion that whatever is intrinsically good is non-instrumentally good. But the converse does not hold. Intrinsic goodness refers to the *moral* sort of what is non-instrumentally good. A common example for something that is non-instrumentally valuable, regardless of any moral consideration, is beauty.

29 This is compatible with the view that something is valuable only if (and because) it is valued by someone.

30 Sometimes a distinction is drawn between *prima facie* harm and all things considered harm (Klocksiem 2012). But to talk of "*prima facie* harm" in this context is misleading. It suggests that something only *appears* to be harmful but is actually not. However, something that is *pro tanto* harmful, *is*, in fact, harmful.

31 Hanser claims that "non-comparatively bad" means "bad for a person [...] regardless of whether a better state was ever a genuine alternative *for him*" (2008, 426).

32 For an overview, see Hanser (2008). Versions of NCA can be found in Shiffrin (2012) and Harman (2004, 2009). Versions of CCA can be found in Feinberg (1986), Parfit (1984), Hanser (2008, 2011), Thomson (2011), Klocksiem (2012), and Feit (2015, 2017). Versions of TCA can be found in Rabenberg (2014) and Zhou (2022).

33 The difference between desire-fulfilment theories and preference-hedonism is that the former appeal to all of our desires about our lives while the latter only appeal to our states of consciousness (see Parfit 1984, 494 and Scanlon 1998, 113).

What about experiential theories or "narrow hedonism"? I follow Parfit (1984, 493) and Scanlon (1998, 113) in rejecting these views. Parfit contends that there is no distinctive common quality of pain or pleasure. What they have in common is their relation to our desires. Prinz makes a similar claim when he argues that the valence of an emotion should be understood as an "inner imperative," such as "more of this!" or "less of this!" (2004, 174). Moreover, as Scanlon (1998, 112) points out, experiential quality is too narrow to assess how well an individual's life is going for them because it makes sense to say that a happy life with false friends is worse for the individual living that life than a happy life with true friends. See also Nozick's (1974) experience machine objection.

34 The distinction between fear and anxiety is understood as follows: "*Fear* is the emotional response to real or perceived imminent threat, whereas *anxiety* is anticipation of future threat" (APA 2013, 189).

35 This does not imply that my fear is something alienated from me.

36 However, it may not give them *sufficient* reason. Especially in health matters, we often think that we should get a second opinion. Nevertheless, it surely gives them a *pro tanto* reason.

References

American Psychiatric Association (APA). 2013. *Diagnostic and Statistical Manual of Mental Disorders: DSM-5*. Arlington: American Psychiatric Association.

Anscombe, Gertrude E. M. 1957. *Intention*. Cambridge, MA: Harvard University Press.

Arpaly, Nomy. 2005. "How It Is Not 'Just Like Diabetes': Mental Disorders and the Moral Psychologist." *Philosophical Issues* 15 (1): 282–298.

Barnes, Elizabeth. 2016. *The Minority Body*. Oxford: Oxford University Press.

Bolton, Derek. 2001. "Problems in the Definition of 'Mental Disorder'." *The Philosophical Quarterly* 51 (203): 182–199.

Boorse, Christopher. 2011. "Concepts of Health and Disease." In *Philosophy of Medicine*, edited by Fred Gifford, 13–64. Munich: Elsevier.

Bortolotti, Lisa. 2013. "Rationality and Sanity: The Role of Rationality Judgments in Understanding Psychiatric Disorders." In *The Oxford Handbook of Philosophy and Psychiatry*, edited by William K. M. Fulford, Martin Davies, Richard Gipps, George Graham, John Sadler, Giovanni Stanghellini, and Tim Thornton, 480–496. Oxford: Oxford University Press.

Bradley, Ben. 2012. "Doing Away with Harm." *Philosophy and Phenomenological Research* 85 (2): 390–412.

Broome, John. 2013. *Rationality through Reasoning*. Malden: Wiley-Blackwell.

Dancy, Jonathan. 2000. *Practical Reality*. Oxford: Oxford University Press.

Davidson, Donald. 1963. "Actions, Reasons, and Causes." *Journal of Philosophy* 60 (23): 685–700.

Dembić, Sanja. 2023. "Mental Disorder: An Ability-Based View." *Philosophy and the Mind Sciences* 4 (2): 1–28.

Edwards, Rem B. 1981. "Mental Health as Rational Autonomy." *Journal of Medicine and Philosophy* 6 (3): 309–322.

Feinberg, Joel. 1986. "Wrongful Life and the Counterfactual Element in Harming." *Social Philosophy and Policy* 4 (1): 145–178.

Feit, Neil. 2015. "Plural Harm." *Philosophy and Phenomenological Research* 90 (2): 361–388.

———. 2017. "Harm and the Concept of Medical Disorder." *Theoretical Medicine and Bioethics* 38 (5): 367–385.

Finlay, Stephen. 2006. "The Reasons That Matter." *Australasian Journal of Philosophy* 84 (1): 1–20.

Foucault, Michel. 1965. *Madness and Civilization: A History of Insanity in the Age of Reason*, trans. Richard Howard. London: Tavistock.

———. 1973. *The Birth of the Clinic: An Archaeology of Medical Perception*. New York: Pantheon Books.

———. 1977. *Discipline and Punishment: The Birth of the Prison*, trans. Alan Sheridan. New York: Pantheon Books.

Gaete, Alfredo. 2008. "The Concept of Mental Disorder: A Proposal." *Philosophy, Psychiatry, and Psychology* 15 (4): 327–339.

Gert, Bernard, Charles M. Culver, and K. Danner Clouser. 2006. *Bioethics: A Systematic Approach* (2nd edn). Oxford: Oxford University Press.

Gibbard, Allan. 2003. *Thinking How to Live*. Cambridge, MA: Harvard University Press.

Gipps, Richard. 2006. "Mental Disorder and Intentional Order." *Philosophy, Psychiatry, and Psychology*, 13 (2). 117–121.

Graham, George. 2010. *The Disordered Mind: An Introduction to Philosophy of Mind and Mental Illness*. London: Routledge.

Gregory, Alex. 2020. "Disability as Inability." *Journal of Ethics and Social Philosophy* 18 (1): 23–48.

Griffin, James. 1986. *Well-Being: Its Meaning, Measurement, and Moral Importance*. Oxford: Clarendon Press.

Hanser, Matthew. 2008. "The Metaphysics of Harm." *Philosophy and Phenomenological Research* 77 (2): 421–450.

———. 2011. "Still More on the Metaphysics of Harm." *Philosophy and Phenomenological Research* 82 (2): 459–469.

Harman, Elizabeth. 2004. "Can We Harm and Benefit in Creating?" *Philosophical Perspectives* 18, 89–113.

———. 2009. "Harming as Causing Harm." In *Harming Future Persons: Ethics, Genetics and the Nonidentity Problem*, edited by Melinda A. Roberts and David T. Wasserman, 137–154. Dordrecht: Springer.

Heinz, Andreas. 2014. *Der Begriff der psychischen Krankheit*. Berlin: Suhrkamp.

Honoré, Antony M. 1964. "Can and Can't." *Mind* 73 (292): 463–479.

Jaster, Romy. 2020. *Agents' Abilities*. Berlin: De Gruyter.

Kiesewetter, Benjamin. 2017. *The Normativity of Rationality*. Oxford: Oxford University Press.

Kittle, Simon. 2015. "Abilities to Do Otherwise." *Philosophical Studies* 172: 3017–3035.

Klocksiem, Justin. 2012. "A Defense of the Counterfactual Comparative Account of Harm." *American Philosophical Quarterly* 49 (4): 285–300.

Kratzer, Angelika. 1977. "What 'Must' and 'Can' Must and Can Mean." *Linguistics and Philosophy* 1 (3): 337–355.

———. 1981. "The Notional Category of Modality." In *Words, Worlds, and Contexts: New Approaches in Word Semantics*, edited by Hans J. Eikmeyer and Hannes Rieser, 38–74. Berlin: de Gruyter.

Lazarus, Richard S. 1991. *Emotion and Adaptation*. New York: Oxford University Press.

———. 1999. "Appraisal, Relational Meaning, and Emotion." In *Handbook of Cognition and Emotion*, edited by Tim Dalgleish and Mick J. Powers, 3–19. Chichester: Wiley.

Leslie, Sarah-Jane. 2007. "Generics and the Structure of the Mind." *Philosophical Perspectives* 21 (1): 375–403.

———. 2008. "Generics: Cognition and Acquisition." *Philosophical Review* 117 (1): 1–47.

Mele, Alfred R. 2003. "Agents' Abilities." *Noûs* 37 (3): 447–470.

Moran, Richard. 2001. *Authority and Estrangement. An Essay on Self-Knowledge*. Princeton: Princeton University Press.

Nordenfelt, Lennart. 1995. *On the Nature of Health an Action-Theoretic Approach* (2nd edn). Dordrecht: Springer.

Nickel, Bernhard. 2016. *Between Logic and the World: An Integrated Theory of Generics*. Oxford: Oxford University Press.

Nozick, Robert. 1974. *Anarchy, State, and Utopia*. Michigan: Basic Books.

Oltmanns, Thomas F., Michele T. Martin, John M. Neale, and Gerald C. Davison. 2012. *Case Studies in Abnormal Psychology* (9th edn). Hoboken, NJ: Wiley.

Parfit, Derek. 1984. *Reasons and Persons*. Oxford: Oxford University Press.

———. 2011. *On What Matters*. Oxford: Oxford University Press.

Prinz, Jesse J. 2004. *Gut Reactions: A Perceptual Theory of the Emotions*. New York: Oxford University Press.

Rabenberg, Michael. 2014. "Harm" *Ethics and Social Philosophy* 8 (3): 1–32.

Railton, Peter. 2003. *Facts, Values, and Norms: Essays Toward a Morality of Consequence*. Cambridge: Cambridge University Press.

Rawls, John. 1971. *A Theory of Justice*. Cambridge, MA: Harvard University Press.

Raz, Joseph. 2009. "Reasons: Explanatory and Normative." In *New Essays on the Explanation of Action*, edited by Constantine Sandis, 184–202. Basingstoke: Palgrave-Macmillan.

Scanlon, Thomas M. 1998. *What We Owe to Each Other*. Cambridge, MA: Harvard University Press.

———. 1993. "Value, Desire, and Quality of Life." In *The Quality of Life*, edited by Martha Nussbaum and Amartya Sen, 185–200. Oxford: Oxford University Press.

Shiffrin, Seanna. 2012. "Harm and Its Moral Significance." *Legal Theory* 18 (3): 357–398.

Stalnaker, Robert C. 2014. *Context*. Oxford: Oxford University Press.

Thomson, Judith Jarvis. 1997. "The Right and the Good." *Journal of Philosophy* 94 (6): 273–298.

———. 2008. *Normativity*. Chicago: Open Court.

———. 2011. "More on the Metaphysics of Harm." *Philosophy and Phenomenological Research* 82 (2): 436–458.

Tremain, Shelley, ed. 2015. *Foucault and the Government of Disability* (2nd edn). Ann Arbor: University of Michigan Press.

———, ed. 2017. *Foucault and Feminist Philosophy of Disability*. Ann Arbor: University of Michigan Press.

Varga, Somogy. 2017. "Mental Disorder Between Naturalism and Normativism." *Philosophy Compass* 12 (6): 1–9.

Velleman, David. 2000. *The Possibility of Practical Reason*. Oxford: Oxford University Press.

Vihvelin, Kadri. 2013. *Causes, Laws, and Free Will: Why Determinism Doesn't Matter*. Oxford: Oxford University Press.

Wolf, Susan. 2010. *Meaning in Life and Why It Matters*. Princeton: Princeton University Press.

Zhou, Yan K. 2022. "What it Means to Suffer Harm." *Jurisprudence* 13 (1): 26–51.

Zimmerman, Michael J., and Ben Bradley. 2019. "Intrinsic vs. Extrinsic Value," in *The Stanford Encyclopedia of Philosophy, edited by* Edward N. Zalta, https://plato.stanford.edu/archives/spr2019/entries/value-intrinsic-extrinsic/.

5 Defending the Rehability View

In this chapter, I defend the Rehability View (RHA) that I presented in Chapter 4. The main arguments for RHA are as follows:

1 RHA meets the adequacy conditions outlined in Section 1.3 to a high degree (assuming that those adequacy conditions are reasonable to begin with).
2 RHA does not face the problems that prevalent views do (see Chapters 2 and 3).
3 RHA can be defended against a couple of objections.

Chapter 5 is structured as follows. In Section 5.1, I address the conceptual distinction between MENTAL HEALTH and MENTAL DISORDER. I demonstrate to what extent RHA meets our actual technical use of "mental disorder" and how it avoids the counterexamples that proved problematic for other views. In Section 5.2, I address the conceptual distinction between MENTAL DISORDER and BODILY DISORDER. In Section 5.3, I address the relationship between having a mental disorder and deviances from social, legal, or moral norms. In Section 5.4, I show how RHA can account for the various normative purposes of the concept MENTAL DISORDER. In Section 5.5, I discuss two possible objections to RHA.

5.1 Mental Health versus Mental Disorder

The first adequacy condition concerns the distinction between MENTAL HEALTH and MENTAL DISORDER. An explication of MENTAL DISORDER (for the purposes described in Section 1.2) should be extensionally adequate in the following sense.
It should include:

1 as many of the overlapping categories of mental disorders listed in the *DSM-5* (APA 2013) and *ICD-11* (WHO 2019) as possible;

DOI: 10.4324/9781003367840-6

2 universal disorders; and
3 the possibility that mental disorders are caused by mechanisms that are spandrels, exaptations, adaptations, or within the normal range of biological functioning.

It should exclude:

4 that (bad, harmful, or unwanted) dispositions (for example, forgetfulness, irritability, timidity, shyness, recklessness, irresoluteness, or laziness) are necessarily mental disorders;
5 typical grief and lovesickness; and
6 homosexuality.

I will explore the extent to which RHA meets the first adequacy condition by discussing these six points in Sections 5.1.1–5.1.6.

5.1.1 Types of Mental Disorder

Ideally, RHA should be able to offer a definition of each type of mental disorder. However, my primary goal is to present a definition of MENTAL DISORDER as a general category rather than definitions of specific types of mental disorder. For this purpose, it suffices to show that RHA can *likely* be employed in formulating specific definitions. In what follows, I describe prevalent types of mental disorders in terms of RHA insofar as the description does justice to what we already know about these metal disorders.[1] I do not contend that these descriptions are sufficient, nor that they are perfectly adequate. They need only be plausible.

1 *Schizophrenia Spectrum and Other Psychotic Disorders*
   S does not have the (non-agentive) ability to not have a certain set of beliefs in view of their mental constitution, a constitution including beliefs that give S sufficient reason against that set of beliefs being true or consistent.

2 *Mood Disorders*
   S does not have the (non-agentive) ability to not be in a certain mood in view of their mental constitution, a constitution that includes beliefs that give S sufficient reason against that mood being objectively adequate.

3 *Anxiety Disorders*
   S does not have the (non-agentive) ability to not experience fear in view of their mental constitution, a constitution that includes beliefs that give S sufficient reason against that fear being objectively adequate.

4 *Obsessive-Compulsive Disorders*
   S does not have the (agentive) ability to not respond with compulsive
   actions to obsessive thoughts in view of their mental constitution, a
   constitution that includes beliefs that give S sufficient reason against
   responding with compulsive actions to obsessive thoughts.

5 *Trauma- and Stressor-Related Disorders*
   S does not have the (non-agentive) ability to not have intrusions in
   view of (1) having experienced a traumatic event and (2) having beliefs
   that give them sufficient reason against these intrusions being objectively adequate (given S's actual situation).

6 *Dissociative Disorders*
   S does not have the (non-agentive) ability to have an "undisrupted
   identity" (in the psychological sense) in view of their mental constitution, a constitution that includes beliefs that give S sufficient reason for
   having a coherent set of beliefs about themselves.

7 *Feeding and Eating Disorders*
   S does not have the (agentive) ability to eat in view of their mental
   constitution, a constitution that includes beliefs that give S sufficient
   reason for eating.

8 *Elimination Disorders*
   S does not have the (agentive) ability to control elimination in view of
   their mental constitution, a constitution that includes beliefs that give
   S sufficient reason to control elimination.

9 *Disruptive, Impulse-Control, and Conduct Disorders*
   S does not have the (agentive) ability to not violate the rights of others or
   major societal norms in view of having beliefs that give them sufficient
   reason against violating the rights of others or major societal norms.
      Or,
   S does not have the (agentive) ability to resist acting on their anger in
   view of having beliefs that give them sufficient reason against acting on
   their anger.

10 *Substance-Related and Addictive Disorders*
   S does not have the (agentive) ability to resist their desire to use some
   substance in view of having beliefs that give them sufficient reason
   against using that substance.

11 *Somatic Symptoms and Related Disorders*
   S does not have the (non-agentive) ability to not have worrying thoughts
   about their somatic symptoms (symptoms that occur without the presence
   of a bodily disorder) in view of their mental constitution, a constitution
   that includes beliefs that give S sufficient reason against those worries.

12 *Paraphilic Disorders*

S does not have the (non-agentive) ability to not have certain paraphilic desires in view of having beliefs that give them sufficient reason against having those paraphilic desires.

Or,

S does not have the (agentive) ability to resist acting on their paraphilic desire in view of having beliefs that give them sufficient reason against acting on their paraphilic desire.

13 *Personality Disorders*

- *Paranoid*: S does not have the ability to trust others in view of having beliefs that give them sufficient reason to trust others.
- *Schizoid*: S does not have the ability to feel attached to others in view of having beliefs that give them sufficient reason to feel attached to others.
- *Schizotypal*: S does not have the ability to feel comfortable with others in view of having beliefs that give them sufficient reason to feel comfortable with others.
- *Antisocial*: S does not have the ability to regard the rights of others in view of having beliefs that give them sufficient reason to regard the rights of others.
- *Borderline*: S does not have the ability to maintain stable relationships with others in view of having beliefs that give them sufficient reason to maintain stable relationships with others.
- *Histrionic*: S does not have the ability to resist being the center of attention in view of having beliefs that give them sufficient reason to resist being the center of attention.
- *Narcissistic*: S does not have the ability to not feel and believe that they are superior to others in view of having beliefs that give them sufficient reason to not feel and believe that they are superior to others.
- *Avoidant*: S does not have the ability to not feel and believe that they are inferior to others in view of having beliefs that give them sufficient reason to not feel and believe that they are inferior to others.
- *Obsessive-Compulsive*: S does not have the ability to release control over how things are going in view of having beliefs that give them sufficient reason to release control over how things are going.

The following types of conditions do not seem to fully fit with RHA. Nevertheless, it is possible to give a rough definition of them that is at least partly in line with RHA.

1 *Neurocognitive Disorders*
S does not have at least one of a certain set of (agentive or non-agentive) cognitive abilities (for example, the ability to sustain attention, remember new information, or recognize emotions in others) in view of their mental or bodily constitution.

2 *Neurodevelopmental Disorders*
S does not have at least one of a certain set of (agentive or non-agentive) cognitive abilities (for example, the ability to reason, learn, communicate verbally, control involuntary actions, or perform actions with focal attention) in view of their mental or bodily constitution.

3 *Sleep–Wake Disorders*
Insomnia: S does not have the (non-agentive) ability to sleep in view of their mental constitution, a constitution that includes arousal, emotions such as anger, worrying thoughts, and unfavorable sleep habits.

4 *Sexual Dysfunctions*
S does not have the (non-agentive) ability to respond sexually in view of their mental constitution.

Let me comment on some of the aforementioned types of conditions.

Neurodevelopmental and Neurocognitive Disorders. The abilities that are impaired in neurodevelopmental and neurocognitive disorders are abilities of φ-ings that are sensitive to reasons (they are cognitive disorders). Nonetheless, the affected individuals do not necessarily lack these abilities in view of their *mental* constitution. Most often, it is in view of their bodily constitution that they lack the requisite cognitive ability. In Alzheimer's, for example, one's bodily constitution may be a certain type of pathological neurological condition. I, therefore, suggest that neurodevelopmental and neurocognitive disorders form a special subset of disorders, one that could be called "somatopsychic" disorders (see Section 5.2).

Sleep–Wake Disorders, Some Sexual Dysfunctions, and Some Somatic Symptom Disorders. Sleeping is neither an action nor a mental state that is sensitive to reasons. Similarly, somatic symptoms such as pain or sexual responses (for example, having an erection) are also not mental states that are sensitive to reasons. However, the individual lacks the relevant abilities in view of their mental constitution. I, therefore, suggest that these types of disorders form another special subset that could be called "psychosomatic" disorders (see Section 5.2).

Personality Disorders. It is common knowledge that the expression "personality disorder" does not literally refer to disorders *of* personality. But what are they disorders of then? Here is a hypothesis. It is striking that almost all personality disorders (except for obsessive-compulsive disorder) concern an individual's relationships to others where the affected individual shows a pattern of behavior that appears largely independent of context (that is, it does not concern relationships to specific individuals but to others quite generally). Thus, one might think of personality disorders as stable but "disordered" ways of dealing with others.

Lastly, let me comment on the *DSM-5* category *gender dysphoria*.

To begin with, it is important to distinguish between "gender dysphoria" and being "trans." An individual experiences gender dysphoria only if they experience affective or cognitive discontent and distress because of the gender assigned to them (see APA 2013, 451). An individual is trans only if the gender assigned to them does not match their gender identity. It is possible that a trans individual does not experience gender dysphoria (at least, not to such an extent that it provides them with a *pro tanto* reason to seek medical, psychiatric, or psychotherapeutic attention). Moreover, it is possible that an individual experiences gender dysphoria but is not trans.

It seems that the *DSM-5* category *gender dysphoria* cannot be adequately captured by RHA. RHA would yield that gender dysphoria is a mental disorder if the definition of "gender dysphoria" were something like the following: S does not have the ability to be affectively or cognitively content with the gender assigned to them in view of their mental constitution, a constitution that includes beliefs that give S sufficient reason for being content with the gender assigned to them.

However, this cannot be a fruitful definition of "gender dysphoria." Individuals experiencing gender dysphoria precisely do not have the (uncontested) belief that the gender assigned to them matches their gender identity (this would give them sufficient reason for being content with the gender assigned to them). On the contrary, they experience cognitive or affective discontent. They believe (at least to some degree) or sense that the gender assigned to them does not match their gender identity.

This is not a flaw in RHA. The fact that an individual experiences gender dysphoria indicates that there is a *mismatch* between their gender identity and the identity assigned to them, and mismatches must be distinguished from disorders. The fact that an individual experiences discontent with the gender assigned to them indicates that their sense of gender does not match the gender assigned to them. And it seems reasonable to assume that gender identity is partly constituted by an individual's sense of gender (see Stoller 1968).

In sum, RHA captures the categories of the *DSM-5* to a high degree and questions the category of "gender dysphoria" as a mental disorder.

5.1.2 Universal Disorders

RHA can capture universal mental disorders. Human beings, in general, have the ability to respond adequately to their available (apparent) reasons in *most* of their reasons-sensitive attitudes and actions (even if we are, of course, unreasonable from time to time). Even individuals with mental disorders generally have the ability to respond adequately to their available (apparent) reasons in most of their reasons-sensitive attitudes or actions. It is just in *some* cases that they lack such an ability. In that sense, their inability is "local" rather than "global." To use Davidson's (1982, 169) words, mental disorder, like irrationality, "is a failure within the house of reason." However, nothing in RHA hinges on how many individuals lack the ability to respond adequately to their available (apparent) reasons in some of their reasons-sensitive attitudes and actions. In fact, it is compatible with RHA that most (or even all) individuals have such local inabilities.

5.1.3 Causal Explanations

RHA has no problem with disorders of spandrels, exaptations, or adaptations. RHA is compatible with the idea that mental disorders can be either caused or constituted by biological mechanisms that fall within the (statistically) normal range of biological functioning. This is because RHA is not committed to any specific causal story of mental disorder. According to RHA, having a mental disorder is a matter of having a certain inability in view of one's mental constitution and one's life circumstances. To have an inability is simply to exhibit a certain *modal pattern* (or a certain modal success rate, see Section 4.2).

RHA is compatible with different views of how to spell out the mental constitution that underlies this pattern. An inability in view of one's mental constitution and one's life circumstances could, for example, result from (a) an impairment (a "broken" or dysfunctional biological mechanism), (b) an underdeveloped biological mechanism, or (c) the fact that the individual's life circumstances constitute too great a burden to bear. To illustrate (c) consider, for example, an individual S who has an addictive disorder when serving as a soldier of war, but no addictive disorder when back at home. RHA can capture the fact that sometimes the relevant change in one's mental constitution, to rid oneself of a mental disorder, can and should be achieved by changing one's life circumstances.

It is worth noting that my claim here is not that one can enable an individual with a mental disorder *without* changing their mental constitution but only that, in principle, changing the individual's mental constitution could also be achieved by changing their external circumstances. Assume that when serving as a soldier of war, S justifiably believes that they live in a stressful environment and that this belief contributes to their addictive disorder. S then returns back home and, thus, changes their external circumstances. Typically, S would thereby also change their mental constitution because they would also stop believing that they live in a stressful environment. If changing S's external circumstances didn't change S's mental constitution, it would be hard to understand how such a change of the external circumstances could have an effect on their mental health.

In sum, RHA puts no restrictions on causal explanations of mental disorders.

5.1.4 Dispositions

(Bad, harmful, or unwanted) dispositions are not necessarily mental disorders. One can, for instance, be timid without having an anxiety disorder or irascible without having an oppositional defiant disorder. RHA can capture this distinction because it explicates MENTAL DISORDER in terms of inabilities, and it excludes dispositions to φ where the φ-ing is not sensitive to reasons to begin with.

How are abilities and dispositions related? This is a matter of dispute. Some argue that abilities are actually a special sort of disposition (for such a view, see Smith 2003; Vihvelin 2004, 2013; Fara 2008; for criticism, see Clarke 2009; Vetter and Jaster 2017; Vetter 2019). There are, though, some interesting similarities and differences that any comprehensive account of the relationship between ABILITY and DISPOSITION must capture (see Jaster 2020, 32). Abilities and dispositions are similar in the following ways:

1 *Instantiation without Manifestation.* Dispositions (for example, a vase's fragility) and abilities (for example, an individual's ability to kill a cat) can both be instantiated without being manifested, that is, one may have a disposition or ability without exercising it. For example, a vase can be fragile without ever breaking, and one can have the ability to kill a cat without ever killing a cat.
2 *Degrees.* Both dispositions and abilities are modal properties that come in degrees. For example, one glass can be more fragile than another (see Manley and Wasserman 2008, 71) and one person can be better at playing the guitar than another (see Jaster 2020, 23).

However, it appears that not all dispositions are abilities. For example, we wouldn't claim that the vase's fragility or a person's irascibility are the vase's or the person's abilities (see Vetter 2019, 202). It is also possible to have a certain ability without having the corresponding disposition. For example, one may have the ability to kill a cat without the disposition to do so (see Millikan 2000, 52).

In light of this, it is clear that abilities and dispositions are not identical. Whatever their exact relation, abilities are not *mere* dispositions (this leaves open the option that abilities are special sorts of dispositions). This suffices to capture the distinctions that are relevant to an explication of MENTAL DISORDER. According to RHA, mental disorders, such as anxiety disorder and oppositional defiant disorder, are defined by an inability to respond adequately to some of their available (apparent) reasons. Plausibly, the forms of timidity and irascibility that we need to exclude are mere dispositions. Let me elaborate on this by discussing a view on which abilities are a special sort of disposition.

According to Jaster (2020, 165), an analysis of ABILITY has a success condition, whereas an analysis of DISPOSITION does not.[2] Jaster spells this out as follows:

SUCCESS$_{\text{ABILITY}}$ An agent S has an *ability* to φ if and only if S φs in a sufficient[ly high] proportion of the relevant possible situations in which some S-trigger for φ-ing is present.

(2020, 165)

DISPOSITION   An object X has a *disposition* to φ if and only if X φs in a sufficient[ly high] proportion of the relevant possible situations in which *some* trigger—in the case of a disposition, a stimulus—for φ-ing is present.[3]

(2020, 164)

Recall that "S-triggers" are triggers, in response to which φ-ing counts as a success (see Section 4.2). In light of SUCCESS$_{\text{ABILITY}}$ and DISPOSITION, one could hold that "abilities are dispositions to φ in response to triggers, in response to which φ-ing counts as a success" (Jaster 2020, 165).

Such a view can capture the relevant dissimilarities. Ascriptions of abilities relate to success, while ascriptions of (mere) dispositions do not. This explains why we would not say that a vase's fragility is an "ability." That a vase breaks when struck is not a success. It also explains the difference between having the ability and the (mere) disposition to kill a cat. An individual S has the ability to kill a cat if and only if S kills a cat in a sufficiently high proportion of the relevant possible situations in which S intends to kill a cat. Given S's intention, killing a cat is a success. By contrast, S has the (mere) disposition to kill a cat if and only if S kills a cat in a sufficiently high proportion of the relevant possible situations in which some trigger (say, a cat) is present. S's ability to kill a cat can be very high (every time they intend to kill a cat, they succeed), but their disposition to do so can concurrently be very low (they almost never have the intention to kill a cat when one is present).

To apply this to a case of non-agentive inability, consider an individual who does not have the ability to digest food. This is a (non-agentive) ability because digesting food is not an action, but it counts as a success in response to ingesting food (it is, after all, the biological function of an individual's digestive system to digest food). On Jaster's Success View, S lacks the (non agentive) ability to digest food if and only if S does not digest food in a sufficiently high proportion of the relevant possible situations in which S ingests food. This is equivalent to claiming that S has the disposition to fail to digest food when ingesting food. So, lacking an ability to φ corresponds to having a disposition to fail to φ when an S-trigger for φ-ing is present.

Now, recall the case of anxiety disorder from Section 4.5. I argued that S has an anxiety disorder only if they do not have the (non-agentive) ability to respond adequately to those beliefs that give them sufficient available (apparent) reason against experiencing fear. In light of the Success View, this is equivalent to the following: S has the disposition to fail to respond adequately to those beliefs that give them sufficient available (apparent) reason against experiencing fear.

How could this clarify the relationship between timidity and anxiety disorder (assuming that DISPOSITION is the correct analysis of what it is to have a disposition)? In both timidity and anxiety disorder, S has a disposition to experience fear. That is, S experiences fear in a sufficiently high proportion of the relevant possible situations in which some trigger is present. However, anxiety disorder differs from timidity along at least three dimensions: (1) which possible situations are *relevant*, (2) what ratio counts as "*sufficient*," and (3) how *intense* S's fear is.

According to RHA, we must evaluate the following three aspects when considering whether an individual S has an anxiety disorder: we must evaluate (i) whether S's fear is inadequate given their epistemic situation, (ii) whether S is able to respond adequately to their beliefs that give them sufficient available (apparent) reason against experiencing fear, and (iii) whether S is harmed by their condition. So, in anxiety disorder, the relevant possible situations are those in which S has beliefs that give them sufficient available (apparent) reason against experiencing fear (so the trigger is an S-trigger). And, both the ratio that counts as "sufficient" and the intensity of the fear will be much higher than in mere timidity. This is because being slightly more afraid and only in a few situations in which one does not have sufficient available (apparent) reason to be afraid is hardly harmful.

When we say that "S is timid," we typically think of S as only slightly more afraid (and, perhaps, afraid in a larger range of situations) than individuals typically are. Moreover, the relevant possible situations to evaluate timidity are not restricted to those in which S's fear is inadequate in light of their epistemic situation. One individual can be more timid than another one even if both have sufficient available (apparent) reason to be afraid. Lastly, timidity need not be harmful to the affected individual.

In sum, anxiety disorder refers to a certain type of *harmful failure*, while timidity (at least, the types we want to exclude from MENTAL DISORDER) is not directly connected to any success or harm condition. In other words, anxiety disorder picks out a special sort of disposition (if abilities are dispositions at all), while timidity picks out a mere disposition.

5.1.5 Grief and Lovesickness

Is RHA better equipped to distinguish between pathological and non-pathological grief or lovesickness than other Harm Views? *Prima facie*, it is not. Heavy losses and breakups seem to cause suffering, some sort of irrationality, and reduced control over one's behavior. But, in RHA, it is ultimately the individual's ability to respond adequately to one's available (apparent) reasons that matter. And, in the case of non-pathological grief or lovesickness, the individual's mental constitution is such that, typically, they easily regain the ability to respond adequately to their available (apparent) reasons after some period of time.

Why should we believe this? Consider a typical case of grief. In such a case, an individual has a normative reason to grieve. After all, they have suffered a significant loss. They also have a reason to hold on to the individual they have lost (we have reason to hold on to things that are of value and that are valuable to us). But they also have a reason to let their lost loved one go (because the loved one cannot be in that relationship anymore). The typical process of grief is responsive to these mixed reasons. Typical grief involves intense and recurring episodes of sadness ("pangs of grief") with intermittent emotions of love, happiness, gratitude, and so on (see Bonanno, Goorin, and Coifman 2008). So, typical grief is not just an emotion. It is a complex phenomenon that involves an "oscillation," of sorts, between different types of emotions, emotions whose function it is to help us come to terms with the loss. Individuals experiencing the typical process of grief generally come to terms with their loss. Thus, the mere fact that an individual experiences the typical oscillating process of grief indicates that they can easily regain the ability to respond to their available (apparent) reasons after some period of time.

Ultimately, RHA allows for a differentiated view. Depending on how narrow or wide one understands "mental constitution" to be (that is, which mental states exactly are included in the extensional set to which "mental constitution" refers to), the grieving or lovesick individual will have (or lack) the ability to omit φ-ing. If we focus on the specific mental states that make up grief or lovesickness, then it turns out that the grieving or lovesick individual, typically, cannot omit φ-ing. But, if we look at their mental constitution more broadly, then the grieving or lovesick individual, typically, can omit φ-ing. Thus, grief and lovesickness are disorders if "mental constitution" is understood very narrowly. However, we should not understand "mental constitution" in such a narrow sense because grief and lovesickness are conditions for which individuals typically have adequate coping mechanisms. But if we understand "mental constitution" in a broader sense, then RHA correctly yields that grief and lovesickness are not mental disorders.

5.1.6 Homosexuality

One might worry that RHA falsely implies that homosexuality is a mental disorder. A critic might argue as follows. To be homosexual is to have sexual desires for those of one's own sex (or gender). Sexual desire is an attitude that is sensitive to reasons because a certain why-question applies to it (see Section 4.3). Now, consider an individual who lives in a society that prescribes the death penalty for homosexuality. It seems that this would give a homosexual individual reason against their homosexual desires. But we should not conclude that they have a mental disorder if they lack the ability to change their sexual desires in light of that reason.

The trouble with this objection is that the fact that there is a death penalty for homosexuality is not a reason against homosexual desire. This is because it would be "the wrong kind" of reason (see Hieronymi 2005, 2013). One does not have a sexual desire for a certain individual because external circumstances are favorable. Considerations showing that it is good or bad for me to have a certain sexual desire in certain circumstances are like considerations showing that it is good or bad to believe something. These considerations do not render the belief rationally intelligible to the believer. Sexual desire is not about external circumstances; it is about a certain individual. Reasons for or against a sexual desire are given by the qualities of "the object" of desire: whether the sexually desired individual is worthy of sexual desire. That there is a death penalty for homosexuality might be a reason not to act on one's homosexual desires, but it is not a reason against homosexual desire itself.

Does RHA yield that homosexuality is a mental disorder? I would argue that it does not. Because it is not the case that objects of homosexual desire are unworthy of such desire simply because they are members of the same sex (or gender). Nothing about the sameness of sex (or gender) justifies such a verdict. However, it is worth noting that this is a substantive claim about values and as such, it might need further argument. Regardless of that, I would like to emphasize that in light of RHA, conflicting views about the status of homosexuality as a mental disorder are conceived of as conflicts about values. As such, they are conflicts that cannot be solved by empirical findings (as biological dysfunction views suggest).

5.2 Mental Disorder versus Bodily Disorder

The second adequacy condition concerns the distinction between MENTAL DISORDER and BODILY DISORDER. In Section 1.3, I pointed out that this distinction might be relevant for both theoretical and practical purposes. We might need an understanding of it to determine the scope of psychopathology and to make a difference for therapeutic purposes. Recall that I am primarily concerned with the conceptual distinction between MENTAL DISORDER and BODILY DISORDER and not with the metaphysical mind-body problem. In addition, I do not need to provide a positive explication of BODILY DISORDER given that my project involves an explication of MENTAL DISORDER.

Most generally, I propose that mental disorders are "mental" in the sense that they *involve* attitudes or actions that are sensitive to reasons. This view is wider than the one I put forward in Chapter 4. However, as noted, RHA should be conceived of as an explication of MENTAL DISORDER for the clearest (types of) cases falling under that concept. My aim here is to widen RHA to include other (types of) cases.

How exactly are attitudes or actions that are sensitive to reasons involved in mental disorder? According to the ability-based view I put forward, for S to have a mental disorder is for S to lack a certain ability to φ, and abilities are always had in view of certain facts. To individuate a certain type of ability we have to specify, at least, two things: (1) the type of φ-ing and (2) the type of facts in view of which we are interested in knowing whether an individual has the ability to φ. On the ability-based view, reasons-sensitive attitudes or actions can then, in principle, be involved in (1) or (2). In the clearest (types of) cases of MENTAL DISORDER, both the φ-ing and the facts are "mental" in the sense that they are attitudes or actions that are sensitive to reasons:

DISORDER$_{PSY}$ An individual S has a DISORDER$_{PSY}$ only if S lacks an ability to φ (where the φ-ing is *mental*) in view of their *mental* constitution, where "mental" refers to attitudes or actions that are sensitive to reasons.[4]

What does the ability-based view tell us about BODILY DISORDER? Not much. It tells us only that "bodily" refers to φ-ings and states that are *not* sensitive to reasons. But this does not give us a positive explication of BODILY DISORDER.

However, since an ability has two aspects (namely, the type of φ-ing and the facts F in view of which the ability to φ is had) that can, in principle, be either bodily or mental, the ability-based view allows for three further disorder-related distinctions:

DISORDER$_{\text{SOM}}$ An individual S has a DISORDER$_{\text{SOM}}$ only if S lacks an ability to φ (where the φ-ing is *bodily*) in view of their *bodily* constitution.

DISORDER$_{\text{PSYSOM}}$ An individual S has a DISORDER$_{\text{PSYSOM}}$ only if S lacks an ability to φ (where the φ-ing is *bodily*) in view of their *mental* constitution.

DISORDER$_{\text{SOMPSY}}$ An individual S has a DISORDER$_{\text{SOMPSY}}$ only if S lacks an ability to φ (where the φ-ing is *mental*) in view of their *bodily* constitution.

DISORDER$_{\text{PSYSOM}}$ and DISORDER$_{\text{SOMPSY}}$ involve attitudes or actions that are sensitive to reasons. Thus, the view that mental disorders are "mental" in the sense that they involve attitudes or actions that are sensitive to reasons implies that DISORDER$_{\text{PSYSOM}}$ and DISORDER$_{\text{SOMPSY}}$ should be considered types of mental disorders. On this quite general view, the category MENTAL DISORDER has three subcategories: DISORDER$_{\text{PSY}}$, DISORDER$_{\text{PSYSOM}}$, and DISORDER$_{\text{SOMPSY}}$.

In light of this, we can formulate a more general view of RHA$_{\text{PSY}}$ (see Section 4.6):

RHA$_{\text{GEN}}$ An individual S has a mental disorder if and only if

i   S does not have the ability to respond adequately (a) to some of their available (apparent) reasons for (or against) some of their reason-sensitive attitudes or actions *or* (b) to something that is no such reason, *in view of* their mental or bodily constitution and their life circumstances (where the threshold of inability is determined by the degree at which individuals in the relevant comparison class are, on average, harmed by their condition C in some respect X) and

ii   S is harmed by their condition C in some respect X, *where X is some component of what makes S's life a non-instrumentally good one for S.*

RHA$_{\text{GEN}}$ includes DISORDER$_{\text{SOMPSY}}$ because it does not confine mental disorder to the inability to respond adequately to one's available (apparent) reasons in view of one's mental constitution. It also includes DISORDER$_{\text{PSYSOM}}$ because it includes inadequate responses to something that is not an available (apparent) reason. Consider the following example of a DISORDER$_{\text{PSYSOM}}$. S lacks the ability to sleep in view of the fact that S worries a lot during the night. Sleeping is not a reasons-sensitive φ-ing because the relevant why-question does not apply to it. Though we can have reasons for or against *going to sleep* (which is an action), we cannot have reasons for or against *sleeping* (which is not an action). This is to say that S's worries are not available (apparent) reasons for S to not sleep. So, by responding to the worries by not sleeping, S responds inadequately to something that is no such reason to begin with. S does not sleep in response to something that they *take* to be reasons against sleeping when they, in fact, are not reasons for not sleeping (not even apparent ones). The adequate response would be to not take the worries to be reasons against sleeping (or to take them to be reasons to solve the problems one worries about).

If one were to apply this view to BODILY DISORDER, it would again suggest that the general category BODILY DISORDER has three subcategories: DISORDER$_{SOM}$, DISORDER$_{PSYSOM}$, and DISORDER$_{SOMPSY}$. On this view, the concepts MENTAL DISORDER and BODILY DISORDER would then overlap. However, I do not settle on this view here, given that this is a top-down proposal (derived from an explication of MENTAL DISORDER). RHA is developed with respect to clear cases of MENTAL DISORDER. But it is open to question whether it can be transferred to cover cases of BODILY DISORDER. Perhaps, there is no one characterization that covers all disorders. To provide an explication of BODILY DISORDER, we have to start with clear cases of bodily disorder and then see how the explications of MENTAL DISORDER and BODILY DISORDER relate to each other. In the following, my modest aim is to explore whether the top-down proposal might be worthy of further pursuit.

Do the aforementioned disorder-related distinctions provide a fruitful categorization of what can generally be called "departures from health"? And, how do they relate to our actual usage? Note that the distinction between DISORDER$_{PSYSOM}$ and DISORDER$_{SOMPSY}$ is similar to the distinction between so-called psychogenic disorders and somatogen disorders (see Schepank 1995). But these distinctions are not equivalent. "Psychogenic" disorders (which are sometimes also called "psychosomatic" disorders) are bodily disorders caused by mental events or processes. "Somatogen" disorders are mental disorders caused by bodily events or processes. But, the DISORDER$_{PSYSOM}$/DISORDER$_{SOMPSY}$ distinction does not make a claim about causes. The "in view of" part of an ability-ascription does not necessarily refer to a causal relation. The role of the "mental" or "bodily" constitution is to "fix" the relevant possible situations needed to evaluate whether an individual has the ability to φ. What causes the respective lack of ability is a different question, one that RHA does not purport to answer.

Prima facie, the provided distinctions do not seem to map onto our actual usage. First, our actual usage of "mental disorder" does not seem to have the tripartite structure suggested earlier (DISORDER$_{SOM}$, DISORDER$_{PSYSOM}$, and DISORDER$_{SOMPSY}$). Second, DISORDER$_{SOM}$, DISORDER$_{PSYSOM}$, and DISORDER$_{SOMPSY}$, taken together, do not seem to map onto our actual usage of "bodily disorder" (or "disease" in the widest sense). However, the matter is a bit more complex. Let me now take a closer look at our actual usage of "mental disorder" and "bodily disorder" in turn.

Mental Disorder. A closer look reveals that we do, in fact, take MENTAL DISORDER to have a tripartite structure, but we capture it using different labels. Consider somatic symptom disorders (which fall under DISORDER$_{PSYSOM}$) and neurodevelopmental and neurocognitive disorders (which fall under DISORDER$_{SOMPSY}$). These are considered mental disorders. Somatic symptom disorders are also called "somatoform" disorders because they involve the presence of somatic symptoms without the presence of a bodily disorder. Neurodevelopmental and neurocognitive disorders are called "neuro-" disorders because they (most often) involve a dysfunction or impairment in the development of the brain or the central nervous system. So, it might be that the suggested tripartite structure of MENTAL DISORDER does map onto our actual usage of "mental disorder." Hence, RHA might provide a fruitful explication of the relevant subcategories.

To clarify matters even more, let me analyze in more detail what RHA yields for somatic symptom disorder. The diagnostic criteria for somatic symptom disorder do not only include the presence of somatic symptoms (without the presence of a bodily disorder). They also include the presence of worrying (or negative thoughts and feelings about the somatic symptoms). This suggests that there are two impairments of abilities involved in somatic symptom disorder: (1) the inability to not have certain somatic symptoms in view of one's mental constitution and (2) the inability to not worry about certain somatic symptoms in view of one's mental constitution. Regarding (1), RHA yields that somatic symptom disorder falls under DISORDER$_{PSYSOM}$. Regarding (2), RHA yields that somatic symptom disorder falls under DISORDER$_{PSY}$.

Does this imply that an individual with a somatic symptom disorder (that includes worrying) actually has two types of disorders? Strictly speaking, yes. But this is not a shortcoming of RHA. RHA does not entail that our classification systems should list every possible type of disorder. An explication of MENTAL DISORDER for normative purposes should yield the conditions that are worthy of psychiatric or psychotherapeutic concern. Whether and how they enter our classification systems should be determined by further practical considerations. For example, if a certain lack of ability almost never gets instantiated, then, for practical reasons, it does not make sense to include that lack of ability as a disorder in our classification systems. Or, if two types of ability impairments are closely related to each other and they are often instantiated together, then it makes sense to cluster them into one category. In somatic symptom disorder, this is exactly the case. The ability-descriptions refer to the same somatic symptoms. Thus, it makes sense to cluster them together into one category.

Bodily Disorder. Do DISORDER$_{\text{SOM}}$, DISORDER$_{\text{PSYSOM}}$, and DISORDER$_{\text{SOMPSY}}$, taken together, map onto our actual usage of "bodily disorder" (or "disease" in the widest sense)? Or, could they provide a fruitful explication of BODILY DISORDER?

There is a crucial difference between mental disorders and bodily disorders, one that suggests that explications of their associated concepts should not be strictly analogous. Mental disorders are ascribed to individuals as a whole and have person-level effects, but bodily disorders need not have person-level effects. They may be restricted to some part or mechanism of an individual. As Boorse puts it, "a small infection, of skin or an internal organ, quickly cured by the immune system, is a self-limiting pathology that may never have gross effects" (2011, 21). This is why the conditions stated in DISORDER$_{\text{SOM}}$ and DISORDER$_{\text{SOMPSY}}$ are not necessary for having a bodily disorder. Moreover, if bodily disorders have person-level effects, then we are prone to consider them (bodily) "disabilities." In fact, taken together, DISORDER$_{\text{SOM}}$ and DISORDER$_{\text{SOMPSY}}$ have some resemblance to Alex Gregory's (2020) analysis of "disability" as "inability." On his view,

> To be disabled is to be less able to do something than is typical, where this degree of inability is partly explained by features of your body that are atypical.
>
> (2020, 26)

Basically, on this view, to be disabled it to be less able to φ (where the φ-ing is either bodily or mental) than is typical in view of one's atypical bodily constitution.

The difference between something having person-level effects versus something not having person-level effects might explain why BODILY DISORDER is, *prima facie*, better explicated by the concept BIOLOGICAL DYSFUNCTION (rather than by the concept INABILITY). This is because the proper bearer of a biological function is a part, process, or mechanism of an organism—that is, a sub-personal entity.

To conclude this section, it appears that the ability-based view does not provide a fruitful explication of BODILY DISORDER. But this is not a shortcoming of RHA. The result just seems to reflect some differences in the phenomena themselves. Mental disorders concern the reasons-sensitive attitudes or actions of individuals as a whole, while bodily disorders concern primarily parts, processes, states, or mechanisms of individuals that are not sensitive to reasons. It should then come as no surprise that the senses in which mental disorders and bodily disorders are "disorders" might differ.

5.3 Mental Disorder versus Deviances from Social, Legal, or Moral Norms

The third adequacy condition concerns the relationship between having a mental disorder and deviances from social, legal, or moral norms. Recall that an explication of MENTAL DISORDER for the purposes described in Section 1.2 should capture the fact that

1 in general, violating a social, legal, or moral norm is neither necessary nor sufficient for having a mental disorder (and *vice versa*), and yet
2 for some types of mental disorders, violations of social, legal, or moral norms play a defining role, and
3 social, legal, or moral norms may play an epistemological role in the diagnosis of some types of mental disorders.

Furthermore, an explication of MENTAL DISORDER should also offer some help in deciding whether

4 we are justified in believing that the worst moral evildoers must have a mental disorder.

1 *Necessity and Sufficiency*
   RHA captures the fact that, in general, violating a social, legal, or moral norm is neither necessary nor sufficient for having a mental disorder. Any lack of an ability to φ (where φ-ing is a reasons-sensitive attitude or action) qualifies as a candidate for a mental disorder (given that the relevant ability is one that individuals generally have and whose diminishment presents a harm to their bearers). Obviously, not all φ-ings that meet these conditions involve social, legal, or moral norms. For instance, being in danger gives me a reason to be afraid, but being in danger is not a moral, legal, or social reason. Thus, RHA captures the fact that violating a social, legal, or moral norm is not necessary for having a mental disorder. Since RHA requires inability (that is, a certain *modal* pattern), it also captures the fact that *actual* violations are not sufficient for having a mental disorder (even in cases in which the type of mental disorder is defined by a type of violation of social, legal, or moral norms).

2 *Defining Role*
   However, there are certain types of φ-ings that do involve social, legal, or moral norms. For instance, individuals, in general, have the ability to refrain from harming the bodily integrity of others in view of having sufficient available (apparent) reasons to refrain from harming the bodily integrity of others. And, "do no harm!" is a moral principle (and

one that is often also legally and socially accepted). So, this ability seems to be defined, partly, by reference to moral norms. This shows that RHA can capture the fact that *some* types of mental disorders can be (partly) defined by reference to social, legal, or moral norms. What, though, justifies our practice of classifying the phenomena that fall under "conduct disorder" as a type of mental disorder? On RHA, we are justified in doing so because individuals are generally able to respond to reasons given by social, legal, or moral norms.

3 *Epistemological Role*

Should having a "bad track record" of violating certain social, legal, or moral norms play an epistemological role in the diagnosis of some types of mental disorders? If we subscribe to RHA, then we should be careful here. According to RHA, one must have a certain inability to have a mental disorder, and abilities are modal properties. An individual's *actual* track record might serve as a kind of heuristic: A "good track record" gives us reason to believe that an individual has the relevant ability to φ because it is evidence of their ability. But, a "bad track record" does not give us reason to believe that the individual lacks the relevant ability to φ. This is because there are several other explanations for why they did not succeed to φ (see Section 4.2). Perhaps, they simply did not try hard enough to φ. So, having a "bad track record" should play only a limited epistemological role (if it plays such a role at all) in the diagnosis of mental disorders. But, then again, what else do we have to evaluate whether an individual *lacks* a certain ability? This highlights the fact that we need an epistemology of abilities (and their limits) that is applicable to the realm of mental disorder.

4 *Worst Moral Evildoers*

Are we justified in believing that the worst moral evildoers have a mental disorder? On RHA, we are not. The mere fact that an individual consistently violates certain social, legal, or moral norms does not show that they do not have the ability to do so. Hence, it is false to assume that the worst moral evildoers necessarily have a mental disorder. Why, then, do we tend to believe that the worst moral evildoers do have a mental disorder? Let me offer two hypotheses.

First, perhaps we simply overgeneralize that an individual's actual behavior figures as a heuristic to their abilities. As already mentioned, a "good track record" gives us reason to believe that an individual has the relevant ability to φ. But a "bad track record" does not give us reason to believe that the individual lacks the relevant ability to φ. Perhaps, we mistakenly assume that the heuristic works in both directions.

Second, the worst moral evildoers act in ways that are so far from what is reasonable given our general mental constitution *qua* human beings that we cannot understand their actions. Perhaps we mistakenly assume that they lack the ability to respond to their available (apparent) reasons because we lack the ability to understand how their actions could possibly be reasonable.

5.4 Normative Purposes

The fourth adequacy condition concerns the fact that we use MENTAL DISORDER for certain normative purposes (see Sections 1.2 and 1.3). We need the concept MENTAL DISORDER to help us settle questions such as (1) whether an individual should seek psychiatric or psychotherapeutic treatment (if available) and (2) whether they should be (partly) exempt or excused from certain social, legal, or moral obligations.

The fact that an individual has a mental disorder provides them with a *pro tanto* reason to seek psychiatric or psychotherapeutic treatment (if available). It also provides others with a *pro tanto* reason to (partly) exempt or excuse that individual from certain social, legal, or moral obligations, or to help them in some way (if possible). An explication of MENTAL DISORDER for these purposes should account for what it is about having a mental disorder that justifies these normative consequences. In the following, I show how RHA can account for the following normative consequences: (1) entitlement to psychiatric or psychotherapeutic treatment, (2) entitlement to sickness benefits, and (3) (partial) exemptions from criminal responsibility.

1 *Psychiatric or Psychotherapeutic Treatment*
According to RHA, an individual is harmed in their having a mental disorder. It is uncontroversial that it is generally a good thing to ameliorate, prevent, or balance harm. Psychiatric or psychotherapeutic treatment aims at (among other things) ameliorating, preventing, or balancing harm. Hence, it is the harm condition in the explication of MENTAL DISORDER that can make intelligible what it is about having a mental disorder that gives the affected individual a *pro tanto* reason to do something to ameliorate their condition. Even more, the concept MENTAL DISORDER can make intelligible why the individual has reason seek to specifically *psychiatric or psychotherapeutic treatment* (if available). This is because in the clearest cases of mental disorder the affected individual is harmed by their low degree of ability to respond adequately to their available (apparent) reasons for some of their *reasons-sensitive attitudes or actions* and in view of their *mental constitution*.

Given that RHA states two conditions for having a mental disorder, I would suggest that psychiatric or psychotherapeutic treatment can have, at least, two aspects: (a) fostering ability (by changing an individual's mental constitution and, in some cases, their life circumstances) and (b) ameliorating harm for the affected individual.

2   *Sickness Benefits*

Treatments of mental disorder can come with significant monetary costs. We can expect (in a statistical sense) that many individuals will get a mental disorder in their lives. Getting a mental disorder is an expectable life risk. The basic idea behind sickness benefits and health insurance is to protect an individual with a mental (or bodily) disorder from financial loss. Who should be entitled to such protection? In short, those who need or have sufficient reason for treatment, but from whom we cannot (in a normative sense) expect to pay (all) the costs. RHA can explain why individuals with mental disorders fall into this group. Some of their abilities are sufficiently impaired, impaired in a way that the individuals are significantly harmed. It is a specific lack of ability that explains why certain normative expectations are not appropriate for individuals who have a mental disorder.

3   *Criminal Responsibility*

Recall that, to be (partly) exempt from criminal responsibility, it is necessary that an individual (a) lacks the ability to understand the difference between what is legally right and wrong or (b) lacks the ability to act in accordance with the understanding of the difference between what is legally right and wrong (see Section 1.2).

For example, Section 20, "Lack of criminal responsibility due to mental disorder," of the German Criminal Code states,

> Whoever, at the time of the commission of the offence, is incapable of appreciating the unlawfulness of their actions or of acting in accordance with any such appreciation due to a pathological mental disorder, a profound disturbance of consciousness or intellectual disability or any other serious mental disorder is deemed to act without guilt.
>
> (Federal Ministry of Justice and Consumer Protection, n.d.)

A forensic psychologist must proceed in three steps when evaluating whether this paragraph applies to an individual.

First, they must evaluate whether the individual in question has (a) a mental disorder ("pathological mental disorder" is a pleonasm), (b) a profound consciousness disorder, (c) intellectual disability, or (d) any other serious mental disorder at the time they performed the unlawful action. "Profound consciousness disorder" includes fatigue, exhaustion, extreme affects, and alcohol-related delirious states.

Second, the forensic psychologist must evaluate whether the individual was (1) able to understand the unlawfulness of their action and (2) able to control (or resist performing) the action *due* to their condition at the time they performed the unlawful action. On the Success View of abilities, we can spell out the criminally relevant abilities as follows:

INSIGHT   At time t, S has the ability to understand the unlawfulness of their action φ if and only if S understands the unlawfulness of φ in a sufficiently high proportion of the relevant possible situations in which (1) all the facts about S's situation are the same as at t and (2) S has beliefs that give them sufficient available (apparent) reason for the unlawfulness of their action φ.

CONTROL   At the time t, S has the ability to resist φ-ing if and only if S resists φ-ing in a sufficiently high proportion of the relevant possible situations in which (1) all the facts about S's situation are the same as at t and (2) S intends to resist φ-ing.

Given RHA, we can see that the inabilities relevant to mental disorder are not identical to the inabilities relevant to (partial) exemptions from criminal responsibility. Consider the following case. S φs and φ-ing is an unlawful action, say, the violation of another individual's basic rights. Assume also that S has a conduct disorder, in the sense that S lacks the ability to omit φ-ing in view of their mental constitution and their life circumstances. Assume further that, at t, S lacks the ability to understand the unlawfulness of φ-ing in view of *all* the facts at t (this will include their mental constitution and life circumstances, but not only, because it will also include all other facts). In this case, the ascribed inabilities are obviously not identical. However, the ascribed inabilities seem to be closely related. In some cases, the mental constitution in view of which S has a conduct disorder might just be the one in view of which S lacks INSIGHT. Having a conduct disorder might (partly) exempt S from criminal responsibility because S's mental constitution might be such that S also lacks INSIGHT.

To conclude this section on RHA, it also becomes clear why having a mental disorder rarely leads to diminished criminal responsibility. None of the characterizations of mental disorder listed in the *DSM-5* or *ICD-11* are defined by (a) a *general* lack of ability to understand the unlawfulness of one's actions or (b) a *general* lack of ability to control one's actions in light of such an understanding (as interpreted in RHA).

5.5 Objections and Replies

In this section, I will consider two objections to RHA and reply to them in turn.

5.5.1 Phenomenal Consciousness Defines the Mental

RHA seems to presuppose that the "mark of the mental"[5] is sensitivity to reasons.[6] However, one might object that the mark of the mental is, instead, phenomenal consciousness (see McGinn 1991; Searle 1992; Strawson 1994). And, not all phenomenally conscious states are states that are sensitive to reasons (for example, sensations such as pain). So, if phenomenal consciousness is the mark of the mental, the objection would go, then the concept of MENTAL DISORDER should not be confined to actions or attitudes that are sensitive to reasons.

I begin my reply by pointing out that RHA does not presuppose that the mark of the mental is sensitivity to reasons. RHA is only committed to the claim that all actions or attitudes that are sensitive to reasons are mental ones. It is not committed to the claim that, metaphysically speaking, *only* actions or attitudes that are sensitive to reasons are mental ones. This is because one might confine the concept of MENTAL DISORDER to actions or attitudes that are sensitive to reasons for other reasons than metaphysical ones. I will now argue that the reason for confining the concept of MENTAL DISORDER in this way is a *practical* one. Let me elaborate.

In medicine, psychiatry, and clinical psychology, merely phenomenally conscious phenomena such as pain do not count as "mental" ones. To see that, consider somatic symptom disorder which is partly defined by an individual having bodily symptoms. A look at the *DSM-5*, the *ICD-11*, and Mathias Berger's textbook on mental disorders (2015, 31 and 536) reveals that the following sets of symptoms typically count as "bodily":

- *Sleep–Wake Symptoms*: insomnia, fatigue, feelings of exhaustion
- *Appetence Symptoms*: hunger, thirst, increase or decrease in libido
- *Gastrointestinal Symptoms*: mouth dryness, heartburn, nausea, vomiting, diarrhea, obstipation, flatulence
- *Cardiorespiratory Symptoms*: breathing problems, coughing, vertigo, palpitation, feeling of pressure in the chest
- *Urogenital Symptoms*: increase or decrease in voiding, unpleasant sensations in the genital area
- *Skin Symptoms*: rubor, bumps, blisters, itching, tingling, burning sensations
- *Pain*: headache, back pain, pain in the limbs, abdominal pain, chest pain
- *Other*: transpiration, shivering, tremor, calor, fever, amenorrhea, tics, bad breath

This set of bodily symptoms comprises bodily changes, some of which come with sensations such as pain, fatigue, itches, tingling, burning sensations, and nausea. (However, not all bodily changes are accompanied by sensations, for example, amenorrhea and certain bumps on the skin).

By contrast, the following sets of symptoms typically count as mental (see Berger 2015, 24 ff.):

- *Attention and Memory*: inattention, distractibility, amnesia
- *Thought*: incoherence, rumination, delusions, suicidal thinking
- *Perception*: illusions, hallucinations
- *Affect (Moods and Emotions)*: depression, hopelessness, guilt, anxiety, flat affect, irritability
- *Behavior*: binge eating, compulsions, stupor, aggressive behavior, self-injurious behavior

The list of bodily and mental symptoms shows that, unlike philosophers, psychiatrists, psychologists, and physicians do not count *sensations* (like pain) as a class of mental phenomena. They also do not count disorders of sensation or of sensory organs (for example, disorders of nociception, blindness, or deafness) as mental disorders. Why this disparity? Perhaps, it is because sensations are merely phenomenally conscious states but not ones that are sensitive to reasons. If this hypothesis is correct, then the mental-bodily distinction in medicine, psychiatry, and clinical psychology is drawn according to whether a certain phenomenon is sensitive to reasons.

The practice of drawing the line between mental and bodily phenomena in virtue of the phenomena's sensitivity to reasons, does not, by itself, count in favor of confining the concept of MENTAL DISORDER to actions or attitudes that are sensitive to reasons. This is because a proponent of the view that phenomenal consciousness is the mark of the mental could argue that this practice reveals an incoherence that should be overcome. However, I will now argue that this practice makes sense, given the normative purposes for which the concept of MENTAL DISORDER should be used (see Section 1.2). Therefore, it makes sense to confine the concept of MENTAL DISORDER in light of this practice.

Confining the scope of psychopathology to phenomena that are sensitive to reasons makes sense because (1) psychiatric and psychotherapeutic treatment (which is not confined to medication) and (2) questions of responsibility make sense only if we are dealing with phenomena that are, in principle, sensitive to reasons. The "talking cure" will not work if my pain is caused by a wound. But, if my pain is caused by a somatic symptom disorder, then exploring whether my attitudes are adequate responses to my available (apparent) reasons might reveal a curative path. Furthermore, I am not responsible for my pain (though I might be responsible for an action of mine that caused my pain). I am, however, responsible for my attitudes and actions which are sensitive to reasons. At least in the sense that

I am *answerable* for them: I can be asked to justify or defend them (see Scanlon 1998 and Smith 2005, 2012). By contrast, it does not make sense to justify or defend my pain.

To conclude, it makes sense to confine the concept of MENTAL DISORDER to actions or attitudes that are sensitive to reasons because these are the phenomena that matter for the normative purposes for which the concept of MENTAL DISORDER should be used. This is a practical reason to confine the scope of psychopathology and not a metaphysical one. We can take this reason into account because we are concerned explicitly with an explication of MENTAL DISORDER for scientific *and* normative purposes.

5.5.2 Harm Is Not Necessary

According to RHA, harm is necessary for having a mental disorder. However, some authors argue that harm is not necessary for having a mental disorder (see Amoretti and Lalumera 2019) or for having a disorder more generally (see Boorse 1997, 2011).

Typical counterexamples to the view that harm is necessary for bodily disorder are minor skin lesions or early stages of certain diseases like prostate cancer (see McGivern and Sorial 2017, 472). Boorse (2011, 51–52) argues as follows. If harm is necessary for having a disorder, and, if being harmed involves being somehow made "worse off," then—contra our actual usage—(1) lower organisms cannot have pathological conditions and (2) there cannot be such a thing as "essential pathology." Referencing Peter Singer (1994, 200), Boorse argues that only beings that have *interests* can be subject to harm (or benefit), and non-sentient beings have no interests. So, if harm were necessary for having a disorder, then beings with no interests could not have a disorder. But we easily ascribe pathological conditions to plants and animals. Boorse also argues that, if one's genotype is essential to one's identity (as for example, Kripke 1980 maintains), then genetic diseases such as Down syndrome cannot make their bearers worse off. This is because the bearer would not have existed without their genetic disease in the first place (see also Kahn 1991; Zohar 1991). Boorse concludes that harm is not necessary for having a disorder.

An obvious counterexample regarding mental disorder is a specific phobia related to spiders in a spider-free environment. Maria Amoretti and Elisabetta Lalumera list further counterexamples (2019, 325–328) such as erectile disorder in an asexual person, schizophrenia in someone who values their hallucinations, minor tics, and early or mild stages of certain disorders (for example, schizophrenia or addictive disorder).

Amoretti and Lalumera (2019) also argue that the *DSM-5* view of harm is problematic. According to them (2019, 322), the harm condition is spelled out in the *DSM-5* in terms of distress or disability. But, as they argue, including the presence of "harm"—in the sense of the presence of distress or disability—as a necessary condition for the presence of a mental disorder produces false negatives (2019, 327). For example, it is possible to have a mild addictive disorder and minor tics without being distressed or disabled (2019, 327–328). On their view, producing false negatives is problematic because many individuals would not be granted entitlements to treatments (because a diagnosis is usually required to be entitled to treatment). This is especially troublesome in cases in which an early diagnosis contains a better prognosis than a later one (2019, 330).

I agree that having a (mental or bodily) disorder in a purely theoretical sense of the term does not require the presence of harm. But, this is not what my project is about. My claim is that harm is necessary for having a mental disorder given an explication of MENTAL DISORDER for (theoretical and) practical or normative purposes. In Section 1.3, I stated that MENTAL DISORDER can help us settle which mental conditions give the affected individual a *pro tanto* reason to seek psychiatric or psychotherapeutic treatment (if available). In Section 5.4, I argued that it is harm that can make intelligible what it is about having a mental disorder that gives the affected individual such a reason. To reiterate, my claim is that having a mental disorder gives the affected individual a *pro tanto* reason to seek psychiatric or psychotherapeutic treatment (if available). This does not imply (a) that the affected individual *should* get psychiatric or psychotherapeutic treatment (if available) nor (b) that *nobody else* has sufficient reason to seek such treatment (if available).

The connection between harm and treatment becomes clear when we consider certain non-pathological conditions, ones that still call for medical attention. Peter Hucklenbroich (2017, 86) offers the following list:

- Discomfort from aging
- Inevitable pain (childbirth, teething, menstruation)
- Gravidity
- Bodily attributes that elicit negative reactions from other individuals or society in general
- Low intelligence or lack of talent
- Mental and emotional problems attributable to difficult life circumstances

Why, though, do these conditions call for medical attention if they are not pathological? Plausibly, because they are (bodily or mental) conditions that are harmful to their bearers.

Thus, my reply to Amoretti and Lalumera's counterexamples is that affected individuals do not have a "mental disorder" in the normatively relevant sense if they are not harmed by their condition. This seems to be correct. For example, if an asexual person with erectile disorder is not harmed by their condition, then they do not have a *pro tanto* reason to seek psychiatric or psychotherapeutic treatment (if available). The same is true of the individual with schizophrenia who values their hallucinations (in case they are not harmed by their condition in any relevant respect).

What about the false-negatives claim? This is an important point. Yet, I do not believe that it presents a problem for my view. Amoretti and Lalumera (2019, 332) themselves point out that the *DSM-5* states that "the fact that some individuals do not show all symptoms indicative of a diagnosis should not be used to justify limiting their access to appropriate care" (APA 2013, 20). As mentioned, my view does not imply that having a mental disorder is the *only* way an individual might have a *pro tanto* reason to seek psychiatric or psychotherapeutic treatment (if available). But why (or in which cases) should individuals with a harmless condition have access to treatment? Why are they deserving of medical concern? Amoretti and Lalumera's (2019, 330) example of early stage cancer suggests an answer: Individuals with a harmless condition should have access to treatment if (1) there is a significant risk of *future harm* and (2) there is reason to believe that there will be benefits from early diagnosis and/or care. If there is not even a risk of future harm, then it is unclear why the condition should be worthy of medical concern. So, even in cases in which there is no actual harm, the concept of HARM can play a role in determining which conditions are worthy of medical concern.

Now, an obvious reply is that my view does not state a necessary condition for having a mental disorder. It suggests only a criterion "to discriminate between mental disorders that must actually be diagnosed or medically treated in practice and mental disorders that need not be" (Amoretti and Lalumera 2019, 332). After all, my view seems to rely on a theoretical concept of MENTAL DISORDER that does not include harm. How else could we ascribe, for example, a harmless erectile *disorder* to an individual? My reply is that we can easily derive a purely theoretical sense of "mental disorder" from RHA$_{PSY}$ if we drop the harm condition.

RHA$_{THEOR}$ An individual S has a mental disorder if and only if S does not have the ability to respond adequately to some of their available (apparent) reasons for (or against) some of their reason-sensitive attitudes or actions; in view of their mental constitution and their life circumstances, (where the threshold of inability is determined by the degree at which individuals in the relevant comparison class are, on average, harmed by their condition C in some respect X, *where X is some component of what makes the lives of these individuals non-instrumentally good ones for them*)

On this view, only abilities to respond adequately to available (apparent) reasons that, when significantly reduced, present a harm to their bearers should be considered pathologies (in a purely theoretical sense). This is the case even if these reduced abilities are, in fact, not harmful to the individual (yet). Only mental conditions that are at least *potentially* harmful to their bearers (in the sense just described) are theoretically interesting. My view captures the fact that we do not classify mental conditions just for the sake of classification. Instead, we do so because mental conditions can have a negative impact on human lives.

Notes

1 Here, I refer to the DSM-5 (APA 2013). For ease of exposition, I shall drop (in Section 5.1.1) "apparent" and "available" when referring to reasons and an individual's "life circumstances" when referring to abilities.
2 To be clear, Jaster does not argue for such an analysis of DISPOSITION. She merely states that this is an "intriguing" (2020, 165) option.
3 There is a debate in the literature on whether dispositionality is a two-place operator—the disposition to M if S—or a one-place operator—the disposition to M—where S is the disposition's stimulus condition, and M its manifestation condition (see Vetter 2015). Vetter (2015) argues that disposition is a one-place operator. If this is correct, then it would suffice to claim that "X φs in a sufficient proportion of the relevant possible situations."
4 This partly corresponds to RHA$_{PSY}$ as described in Chapter 4. Here, I give it a new name to highlight the conceptual distinctions that are relevant in this section.
5 The expression "the mark of the mental" is used to denote the set of necessary and sufficient conditions for something to be mental.
6 This view relates in important ways to the view that intentionality is the mark of the mental (see Brentano 1924; Tye 1995; Dretske 1995; Crane 1998). However, these views are not necessarily identical. Intentionality is the property of many (or perhaps all) mental states to be *about* or *directed towards* something. As such, intentionality is a relational property: a property that relates its bearer to that which the intentional state is about or to a content. By contrast, to be "sensitive to reasons" means that it makes sense to ask a certain question "why?" with respect to certain states (see Section 4.3). Arguably, only intentional states can be sensitive to reasons. But, perhaps, not all intentional states are states that are sensitive to reasons (for example, perceptions).

References

American Psychiatric Association (APA). 2013. *Diagnostic and Statistical Manual of Mental Disorders: DSM-5*. Arlington: American Psychiatric Association.
Amoretti, Maria C., and Elisabetta Lalumera. 2019. "Harm Should Not Be a Necessary Criterion for Mental Disorder: Some Reflections on the DSM-5 Definition of Mental Disorder." *Theoretical Medicine and Bioethics* 40: 321–337.
Berger, Mathias, ed. 2015. *Psychische Erkrankungen. Klinik und Therapie* (5th edn). Munich: Elsevier.

Bonanno, George A., Laura Goorin, and Karin G. Coifman. 2008. "Sadness and Grief." In *The Handbook of Emotion*, edited by Lisa Feldman Barrett, Michael Lewis, and Jeannette M. Haviland-Jones, 797–810. New York: Guilford Press.

Boorse, Christopher. 1997. "A Rebuttal on Health." In *What Is Disease?*, edited by James M. Humber and Robert F. Almeder, 1–134. Totowa, NJ: Humana Press.

———. 2011. "Concepts of Health and Disease." In *Philosophy of Medicine*, edited by Fred Gifford, 13–64. Munich: Elsevier.

Brentano, Franz. 1924. *Psychologie vom empirischen Standpunkt* (2 vols). Leipzig: Felix Meiner.

Clarke, Randolph. 2009. "Dispositions, Abilities to Act, and Free Will: The New Dispositionalism." *Mind* 118: 323–351.

Crane, Tim. 1998. "Intentionality as the Mark of the Mental." In *Royal Institute of Philosophy Supplement*, edited by Tim Crane, 229–251. Cambridge: Cambridge University Press.

Davidson, Donald. 1982. "Rational Animals." *Dialectica* 36 (4): 317–328.

Dretske, Fred. 1995. *Naturalizing the Mind*. Cambridge, MA: MIT Press.

Fara, Michael. 2008. "Masked Abilities and Compatibilism." *Mind* 117: 843–865.

Federal Ministry of Justice and Consumer Protection. n.d. "German Criminal Code." Accessed April 3, 2023. http://www.gesetze-im-internet.de/index.html.

Gregory, Alex. 2020. "Disability as Inability." *Journal of Ethics and Social Philosophy* 18 (1): 23–48.

Hieronymi, Pamela. 2005. "The Wrong Kind of Reason." *Journal of Philosophy* 102 (9): 437–457.

———. 2013. "The Use of Reasons in Thought (and the Use of Earmarks in Arguments)." *Ethics* 124: 114–127.

Hucklenbroich, Peter. 2017. "Disease Entities and the Borderline Between Health and Disease: Where Is the Place of Gradations?" In *Vagueness in Psychiatry*, edited by Geert Keil, Lara Keuck, and Rico Hauswald, 75–92. Oxford: Oxford University Press.

Jaster, Romy. 2020. *Agents' Abilities*. Berlin: De Gruyter.

Kahn, Jeffrey P. 1991. "Genetic Harm: Bitten by the Body That Keeps You?" *Bioethics* 5 (4): 289–308.

Kripke, Saul A. 1980. *Naming and Necessity*. Cambridge, MA: Harvard University Press.

Manley, David, and Ryan Wasserman. 2008. "On Linking Dispositions and Conditionals." *Mind* 117 (465): 59–84.

McGinn, Colin. 1991. *The Problem of Consciousness: Essays Towards a Resolution*. Cambridge: Blackwell.

McGivern, Patrick, and Sarah Sorial. 2017. "Harm and the Boundaries of Disease." *Journal of Medicine and Philosophy* 42: 467–484.

Millikan, Ruth G. 2000. *On Clear and Confused Ideas*. Cambridge: Cambridge University Press.

Scanlon, Thomas M. 1998. *What We Owe to Each Other*. Cambridge, MA: Harvard University Press.

Schepank, Heinz. 1995. "Psychisch versus Psychogen. Eine notwendige Begriffsklärung." *Zeitschrift für Psychosomatische Medizin und Psychoanalyse* 41 (2): 101–107.

Searle, John R. 1992. *The Rediscovery of the Mind*. Cambridge, MA: MIT Press.

Singer, Peter. 1994. *Ethics*. Oxford: Oxford University Press.

Smith, Angela M. 2005. "Responsibility for Attitudes: Activity and Passivity in Mental Life." *Ethics* 115 (2): 236–271.

———. 2012. "Attributability, Answerability, and Accountability: In Defense of a Unified Account." *Ethics* 122 (3): 575–589.

Smith, Michael. 2003. "Rational Capacities, or: How to Distinguish Recklessness, Weakness, and Compulsion." In *Weakness of Will and Practical Irrationality*, edited by Sarah Stroud and Christine Tappolet, 17–38. Oxford: Oxford University Press.

Stoller, Robert J. 1968. *Sex and Gender. The Development of Masculinity and Femininity*. London: Kamac Books.

Strawson, Galen. 1994. *Mental Reality*. Cambridge, MA: MIT Press.

Tye, Michael. 1995. *Ten Problems of Consciousness: A Representational Theory of the Phenomenal Mind*. Cambridge, MA: MIT Press.

Vetter, Barbara. 2015. *Potentiality*. Oxford: Oxford University Press.

———. 2019. "Are Abilities Dispositions?" *Synthese* 196: 201–220.

Vetter, Barbara, and Romy Jaster. 2017. "Dispositional Accounts of Abilities." *Philosophy Compass* 12 (8): 1–11.

Vihvelin, Kadri. 2004. "Free Will Demystified: A Dispositionalist Account." *Philosophical Topics* 32: 427–450.

———. 2013. *Causes, Laws, and Free Will. Why Determinism Doesn't Matter*. Oxford: Oxford University Press.

World Health Organization (WHO). 2019. *International Classification of Diseases 11th Edition (ICD-11)*. Geneva: World Health Organization.

Zohar, Noam J. 1991. "Prospects for 'Genetic Therapy': Can a Person Benefit from Being Altered?" *Bioethics* 5 (4): 275–288.

6 Case Study

Addictive Disorder

In Chapters 4 and 5, I have presented and defended the Rehability View (RHA) as an explication of MENTAL DISORDER. In this chapter, my aim is to illustrate RHA with an example and, by doing so, to demonstrate RHA's fruitfulness. I will present a definition of the concept ADDICTIVE DISORDER in light of RHA. The chapter is structured as follows.[1] In Section 6.1, I propose two adequacy conditions for explicating ADDICTIVE DISORDER. In Section 6.2, I present an explication of ADDICTIVE DISORDER in light of RHA. In Section 6.3, I show how the explication meets the aforementioned adequacy conditions. In Section 6.4, I discuss a competing view put forward by Walter Sinnott-Armstrong and Hanna Pickard (2013). In the final section, I draw some conclusions.

6.1 Adequacy Conditions

An explication of ADDICTIVE DISORDER should capture and clarify:

1 the distinction between addictive disorder and other *similar* types of mental disorders (such as obsessive-compulsive disorder, OCD) and
2 the distinction between *disorder* and *non-disorder*.

This list is not exhaustive, of course. But I focus on these issues because they are troublesome for certain competing views. Let me elaborate on each of these adequacy conditions in turn.

1 *Addictive and Other Similar Types of Mental Disorders*
Individuals with an addictive disorder are sometimes said to be "compelled" to do what they are addicted to doing; it appears that they are in some sense "dependent" on the activity. But there are other types of disorders where the same seems true, for example, OCD. And, yet, addictive disorder and OCD are viewed as two separate types of mental

DOI: 10.4324/9781003367840-7

disorder (APA 2013, 235 and WHO 2019, F42). Hence, an explication of ADDICTIVE DISORDER should capture and clarify the distinction between addictive disorder and other similar types of disorders such as OCD.

2 *Disorder and Non-disorder*
Consider an individual who occasionally drinks alcohol. Obviously, they are not necessarily addicted to alcohol. Even the harmful habit of drinking alcohol must be distinguished from an alcohol use disorder (see Section 5.1). Therefore, an explication of ADDICTIVE DISORDER should capture and clarify the difference between disordered and non-disordered φ-ings.

6.2 The Rehability View of Addictive Disorder

I propose the following explication of ADDICTIVE DISORDER:

AD   An individual S has an addictive disorder if and only if

    i   S recurrently and sufficiently frequently has the desire to φ;
    ii   φ-ing has the potential to cause tolerance or withdrawal;
    iii   S lacks the ability to omit φ-ing in view of their mental constitution and their life circumstances; and
    iv   S is *pro tanto* harmed by φ-ing or their desire to φ.

According to AD, an individual has an alcohol use disorder if and only if they have the desire to drink alcohol recurrently and sufficiently often; they lack the ability to stop drinking alcohol in view of their mental constitution and life circumstances; they are harmed by their alcohol consumption and/or their desire to drink alcohol. Moreover, alcohol consumption qualifies as a candidate for AD because it has the potential to cause tolerance or withdrawal. Since AD provides only an explication of the concept—and not a comprehensive theory—of addictive disorder different views of desire, tolerance and withdrawal, abilities, and harm may yield different verdicts as to which phenomena fall under AD.

Before moving on, let me consider how AD relates to the diagnostic—that is, epistemic—criteria for (substance-related) addictive disorders in the *DSM-5*. According to the *DSM-5* (APA 2013, 481 f.), a problematic pattern of substance use should count as an addictive disorder only if it leads to clinically significant impairment *or* distress, as manifested by at least two of eleven criteria (mild: two to three, moderate: four to five, severe: six or more symptoms) that are grouped into four categories: "impaired control over substance use" (one to four), "social impairment" (five to seven), "risky use" (eight to nine), and "pharmacological criteria" (ten to eleven). AD suggests a slightly revisionary view. Because it takes both inability *and* harm to be necessary, it would require that at least one of the two criteria should be among one to four and ten ("impaired control over substance use" and "tolerance"; tolerance makes resistance more difficult, suggestive of why it may be indicative of the inability to omit substance use), and the other among five to nine and eleven ("social impairment," "risky use," and "withdrawal"; withdrawal is a highly unpleasant experience and counts as "harm").[2] Accordingly, AD is slightly more restrictive than the current practice.

6.2.1 Desire

For an individual to be addicted to φ-ing, it is necessary that they have a desire to φ.[3] I will use "desire" in a wide sense so that it includes wanting, seeking, needing, having an appetite for, craving, or any other motivational state.[4] The desire to φ does not need to be unusually strong. It may be so only relative to an individual's other desires, which may be unusually low in intensity. In addictive disorder, the desire to φ is typically pleasure-seeking, at least in the beginning.[5] From a phenomenological perspective, "feeling better" can be achieved by gaining pleasure or relief (see Hübl 2010, 188); that is, some desires are pleasure-seeking (for example, the desire for chocolate), others are relief-seeking (for example, the urge to urinate or wanting a conference presentation to be over). Relief-seeking desires are about avoiding an expected displeasure or the expected relief from displeasure (wanting the pain to go away). However, as Sinnott-Armstrong and Pickard (2013, 854) highlight, in addictive disorder, the desire to φ may eventually detach from the experience of pleasure when engaging in φ-ing.[6] At this point, the pleasure-seeking desire has become a relief-seeking one. It is worth noting that the desire to φ may simultaneously be both, pleasure- and relief-seeking. For instance, φ-ing may provide some pleasure and relieve the individual from the burden of everyday life.

Condition (1) is not sufficient for having an addictive disorder. If it were, any habitual desire whatsoever (for example, to take a shower) would constitute an addictive disorder.

6.2.2 Tolerance and Withdrawal

The second condition reflects the view that it is not possible for an individual to become addicted to just about anything. Why not? Given the ordinary meaning of the phrase "being addicted to"—which roughly translates as "being dependent on"—all possible φ-ings seem to qualify as candidates for an addictive disorder.[7] We may say that S "is addicted to" watching television series, eating chips, using social media, or any other behavior. However, this view is problematic from a psychiatric perspective because certain φ-ings might be considered addictive when they should not be considered such, either because they are not pathological to begin with (breathing) or because they seem to constitute a pathological condition of a different type (OCD).[8] Humans are dependent on breathing but not addicted to it. Both individuals with OCD and individuals with an addictive disorder appear to be dependent on their behavior. But compulsions in OCD are typically repetitive responses to obsessive thoughts driven by anxiety, whereas substance use in addictive disorder does not typically hinge on such repetitive responses to obsessive thoughts. Thus, not all types of dependency mark a disorder, and not all disordered types of dependencies amount to an addictive disorder.

A glimpse at the empirical literature suggests that the possible φ-ings should be restricted by way of their relation to tolerance and withdrawal.[9] "Tolerance" denotes the decrease of the effectiveness of a substance X after repeated consumption (see Berger 2015, 250). S develops tolerance with respect to a substance X (or any φ-ing) only if the following is true: S would have to use a higher dose of X (or φ more) to attain the same effect as before with a lower dose of X (or with less φ-ing). The concept of withdrawal, however, is less clear. Typically, withdrawal is characterized in relation to the concept of substance. According to the WHO, a withdrawal state is a group of symptoms occurring with the "cessation or reduction of use of a psychoactive substance that has been taken repeatedly, usually for a prolonged period and/or in high doses."[10] But this definition is too narrow because it excludes by definition *all* non-substance-related φ-ings.

Here is a different way of viewing it. Only the individual's negative responses to the cessation of the φ-ings with respect to which they develop tolerance in the first place should be considered "withdrawal symptoms." This view is supported by neurobiology (see Heinz 2014, 2017). Consider alcohol, which has a sedative effect. Regular consumption of alcohol leads to a neurological adaption: the receptors for inhibitory neurotransmitters are downregulated (see Heinz and Batra 2003 and Heinz et al. 2012). This mechanism prevents further potentially life-threatening sedation, which leads to the consequence that an individual can consume more alcohol without becoming more sedated (or in other words, "tolerance"). A cessation of alcohol use leads to a neurological imbalance between inhibitory and excitatory neurotransmitters in favor of the latter because it takes time to upregulate the inhibitory receptors (see Heinz and Batra 2003). Accordingly, the individual experiences various forms of overexcitation (in other words, "withdrawal symptoms"). Such a definition of withdrawal is valuable because it is developed with respect to the paradigmatic cases of addictive disorder while not being restricted solely to them.

However, conditions (1) and (2) are not sufficient for having an addictive disorder. Consider a smoker who experiences anxiety when they stop. They are not necessarily addicted to smoking. If they are perfectly able to stop, then they are simply a non-disordered smoker and would not appear to need psychiatric or psychotherapeutic treatment.

6.2.3 Harm

According to AD, having an addictive disorder necessarily involves harm.[11] Recall the contrast between "harm" and "living a good life," where "living a good life" is as an overarching term for all things that make an individual's life a non-instrumentally good one for the individual who lives it.

Recall also the distinction between *pro tanto* and *all things considered* harm. The inability to omit using substance X may be *pro tanto* harmful to an individual, but all things considered, beneficial. Imagine an individual who uses a substance to alleviate chronic pain owing to a fatal disease. We can easily imagine a context in which we would consider them addicted but still judge that they should keep on using the substance because it is, all things considered, beneficial to them. In any case, AD does not require that the individual is all things considered, only that they are *pro tanto* harmed by φ-ing or their desire to φ. That is, they are harmed by it in some respect X, where X is some component of what makes the individual's life non-instrumentally a good one (for the individual who lives it).

We might ask: why is condition (iv) necessary for having an addictive disorder? Consider the following scenario. Suppose chips fulfilled condition (ii), that is, suppose that chips had the potential to cause tolerance (one would need to gradually increase consumption of them to get the same satisfaction as before) and withdrawal symptoms (one would feel painfully hungry once one quits eating them). Furthermore, suppose that chips had almost no harmful effects. We would probably say—in a colloquial (but also theoretical) sense—that the individual is "hooked" on them. But we would probably not say that they have an "addictive disorder" in the psychiatric, psychotherapeutic, and practical sense because eating chips would not give them a *pro tanto* reason to seek psychiatric or psychotherapeutic treatment. We would not advise them to do anything about their condition, nor would we include the condition in our diagnostic manuals. Though their condition may be considered an "addiction" in a colloquial or purely theoretical sense, this classification would be of no practical relevance.

6.2.4 Inability

The inability condition requires more elaboration than the other conditions. Consider two individuals that engage in the same behavior, for example, drinking beer. There is a difference between an individual who drinks beer and has an alcohol use disorder and an individual who drinks beer but does not have such a disorder. According to AD, the difference is that the former lacks the ability to omit drinking alcohol in view of their mental constitution and life circumstances, whereas the latter has that ability.

To elaborate on this condition, recall Jaster's Success View of agentive abilities:

SUCCESS$_{AA}$ S has an agentive ability to perform an action φ if and only if S φs in a sufficiently high proportion of the relevant possible situations in which S intends to φ (where the set of the relevant possible situations will vary across ascriber contexts).

(2020, 98 and 159)

According to AD, the relevant possible situations are those in which the individual's mental constitution and their life circumstances are held fixed. "Mental constitution" and "life circumstances" are vague concepts: they refer to an individual's relatively stable attitudes and external circumstances (see Section 4.2).

Why should we believe that these factors are relevant? On the one hand, it is clear that we should not abstract from the individual's *desires*, because an individual with an addictive disorder may well have the ability to omit φ-ing if they did not have the desire to φ. But this ability does not make them any less of an addict. The same appears to be the case with their other, more stable attitudes. For the purposes of diagnosis, we want to know whether *this* particular individual has the ability to omit φ-ing and not whether they would have the ability to omit φ-ing if they were a different person. On the other hand, we should abstract from certain volatile mental states. An individual may lack the ability to omit φ-ing in view of their current euphoric mood, but on its own, this does not count toward having an addictive disorder. The same reasoning applies to an individual's external circumstances: we should not abstract from the individual's general life circumstances. They may have the ability to omit φ-ing if their external circumstances were wholly better, and yet this ability does not make them any less of an addict. We should, however, abstract from the more volatile external circumstances; once in a while we all get into tempting circumstances in which we fail to omit φ-ing, but these failures do not necessarily count against our abilities to omit φ-ing.

What is the standard of sufficiency? In light of RHA (see Section 4.2), the threshold of inability in the case of addictive disorder is determined by the degree at which the individuals in the relevant comparison class are, on average, harmed by φ-ing or their desire to φ.

One benefit of explicating the inability condition in terms of the Success View is that it can capture a broader perspective wherein an addict's inability to omit φ-ing may be located on different levels. Let me elaborate.

The Success View can deal with cases of so-called impeded intentions. Consider Betty, a golfer currently in a coma (see van Inwagen 1983, 11). There is a good sense in which Betty "cannot" play golf; she cannot even form the intention to play golf to begin with. SUCCESS$_{AA}$ can capture these cases correctly, because it is not true that Betty plays golf in a sufficiently high proportion of the relevant possible situations in which she is in a coma and intends to play golf. Why not? Because there are no relevant possible situations in which she is in a coma *and* also intends to play golf. Thus, the modal success ratio is either unspecified or zero (see Jaster 2020, 109). The SUCCESS$_{AA}$ correctly yields that Betty lacks the ability to play golf because, either way, modal success ratio in this case is certainly not sufficiently high. More generally, SUCCESS$_{AA}$ entails that there is a relevant possible intention situation to begin with (see Jaster 2020, 109). If S cannot form the intention to φ to begin with, SUCCESS$_{AA}$ correctly yields that S, *a fortiori*, does not have the ability to φ.

There may be similar cases in addictive disorder. Imagine an individual with an addictive disorder who lacks the ability to form the intention to omit φ-ing to begin with (perhaps they have conflicting desires, while the desire to continue φ-ing always prevails). If the individual lacks the ability to form the intention to omit φ-ing to begin with, there is obviously a sense in which they lack the ability to omit φ-ing. SUCCESS$_{AA}$ captures these cases in the same way it captures cases in which an individual is in a coma.

One might object that the problem of real-world individuals with an addictive disorder does not really rest on the level of forming intentions, or that this clinical group is insignificant. It is, however, important to distinguish between empirical and conceptual questions. It is an empirical question whether and, if so, what proportion of the individuals with an addictive disorder lack the ability to form the intention to omit φ-ing to begin with. Although it seems implausible to assume that there are individuals with an addictive disorder in the actual world who cannot form a *desire* to omit φ-ing, it is more plausible to assume that there are such individuals who cannot form the *intention* to omit φ-ing. Intentions are supposed to resolve conflicting desires. Because of that, having an intention to omit φ-ing requires more than simply having a pro-attitude toward the omission of φ-ing; it requires a commitment to omit φ-ing. Imagine an individual with equally strong desires that are in conflict with each other, someone who just cannot "make up their mind." Any "commitment" worthy of the name will need to prevail in at least some of the situations in which one is tempted to φ. But, given the structure of addictive desires, this precisely is the problem. It is a common feature of human psychology that the future effects are discounted in the face of present rewards. But in addictive disorder, discount curves are typically hyperbolic: the closeness of the reward of φ-ing sharply increases its value so that the future potential reward of omitting φ becomes relatively low (see Ainslie 2000 and Heyman 2009). Thus, it is not clear that the clinical group of individuals with an addictive disorder whose problem is concerned with an inability to form intentions to begin with is insignificant.

Furthermore, even if the clinical group were insignificant, it would not follow that their condition does not fall under ADDICTIVE DISORDER. No matter how small the set of empirical cases, a definition should not yield that some of the worst imaginable cases of addictive disorder—an individual who cannot even form the intention to omit φ-ing to begin with—are excluded from the extensional set of ADDICTIVE DISORDER.

However, cases of addictive disorder differ from coma cases in one crucial respect. Whereas Betty cannot form intentions *tout court*, individuals with an addictive disorder, if at all, cannot form *certain* intentions. I propose that if the individual's problem is at the level of intention, then it is the ability to form specifically *rational* intentions that matters most.[12] Jaster does not offer an analysis of this ability, but with her view in hand, I propose the following analysis:

SUCCESS$_{RI}$ S has the ability to *rationally intend* to φ if and only if S intends to φ in a sufficiently high proportion of the relevant possible situations in which S judges to have decisive reason to φ (where the set of the relevant possible situations will vary across ascriber contexts).

In light of this, we can see that, in principle, an addict may also have a problem at an even more fundamental level, namely, that of judgment. Here is an analysis for that ability:

SUCCESS$_{J}$ S has the ability to *judge* that they have decisive reason to φ if and only if S judges that they have decisive reason to φ in a sufficiently high proportion of the relevant possible situations in which S is presented with decisive reason to φ (where the set of the relevant possible situations will vary across ascriber contexts).

In sum, an individual's inability to omit φ-ing may be located on different levels. First, an individual may have the ability to intend to omit φ-ing but lack the ability to *follow through* with their intentions. Second, an individual may lack the ability to *form a rational intention* to omit φ-ing to begin with (that is, they may lack the ability to form an intention to omit φ-ing in response to their judgment that they have decisive reason to omit φ-ing). Third, an individual may lack the ability to *form a judgment* that they have decisive reason to omit φ-ing when presented with such reasons.

6.3 Meeting the Adequacy Conditions

In this section, I show how AD can meet the adequacy conditions proposed in Section 6.1.

6.3.1 Addictive Disorder and Other Similar Types of Disorders

AD helps to pinpoint the difference between addictive disorder and other similar types of disorders by clarifying the dimensions of (dis-)similarity. In light of AD, addictive disorder is similar to OCD in that both definitions include conditions (i), (iii), and (iv): desire, ability, and harm. But addictive disorder differs from OCD with respect to the dimension delineated in condition (ii), namely the type of φ-ing at stake. In light of AD, OCD differs from addictive disorder in that the types of φ-ing involved in OCD—compulsions such as repetitive handwashing—do not typically have the potential to cause tolerance and withdrawal.

Let me make two clarifications. First, AD does not entail that there are no other relevant differences between addictive disorder and other similar types of disorders. There might be other differences, with respect to the phenomenology of a desire or the type of harm, for example. Addictive disorder typically begins with pleasure-seeking desires. By contrast, OCD typically begins with relief-seeking desires, and the φ-ing has the potential to cause relief from displeasure owed to obsessive thoughts (but not the potential to cause pleasure). However, as mentioned in Section 6.2.1, desires in addictive disorder can become relief-seeking. Furthermore, the displeasure caused by addictive φ-ing may, in principle, manifest itself in the form of obsessive thoughts (which center on φ-ing). So, distinguishing between addictive disorder and OCD in terms of the various types of desire involves some fuzziness.

Now, a similar problem emerges in connection with tolerance and withdrawal. What if someone with OCD has to φ, but this activity gradually increases in frequency because they experience panic when not φ-ing. Does this not sound like the experience of tolerance and withdrawal? Furthermore, there seems to be a connection between pleasure-seeking desires in addictive disorder and tolerance: tolerance is a "safety-mechanism" of the organism that prevents any potentially life-threatening effects of the substances causing pleasure. So, again, the distinction involves some fuzziness.

In this regard, we can spell out the differences in two directions: in terms of tolerance and withdrawal, or in terms of pleasure-seeking versus relief-seeking desires. But neither distinction will be sharp; both involve a degree of fuzziness. Perhaps fuzziness is unavoidable because the phenomena we seek to grasp in our categories of "addictive disorder" and "OCD" are not so neatly sorted. We can, however, still point to some *typical* characteristics. Addictive disorders typically involve φ-ings that have the potential to cause tolerance and withdrawal and typically do not involve obsessive thoughts and repetitive φ-ings. By contrast, OCD typically involves φ-ings that have the potential to cause relief from displeasure owed to obsessive thoughts and typically does not involve φ-ings that have the potential to cause tolerance and withdrawal.

Moreover, AD does not imply that all cases meeting conditions (i), (iii), and (iv) are cases of OCD *unless* they meet condition (ii). Rather, the phenomena captured by conditions meeting conditions (i), (iii), and (iv) constitute the broad class of "agentive disorders," two of which are OCD and addictive disorder. But there may be countless other types of agentive disorders (for example, eating disorders). Again, these can be differentiated by their characteristic φ-ings. The φ-ing in OCD is a repetitive behavior in response to obsessive thoughts, whereas the φ-ing in addictive disorder has the potential to cause tolerance and withdrawal (the φ-ing in eating disorders appears to diverge from both).

AD can also capture the possibility of subtypes of addictive disorder, again by way of condition (ii). Any type of φ-ing that has the potential to cause tolerance or symptoms of withdrawal qualifies as a subtype of addictive disorder. In this connection, it may be argued that gambling is similar to substance use. Consequently, whether the inability to omit exercising, having sex, or shopping qualifies these activities as subtypes of addictive disorders (rather than as other types of mental disorders) depends on whether they have the potential to cause tolerance or withdrawal symptoms in the same way that substance use (and gambling) does.

Let me now reply to a potential objection. Imagine an individual with a pattern of substance use that looks exactly like addictive disorder, except that the substance does not have the potential to cause tolerance or withdrawal. Wouldn't we still count them as having an addictive disorder? All things being equal, I believe that we would. And yet this does not refute AD because condition (ii) is decidedly empirical. This is to say that, for all we know, the phenomena we subsume under the label "addictive disorder" have, *as a matter of fact*, a common trait, which is that φ-ing has the potential to cause tolerance and withdrawal. What the hypothetical case shows is that our ordinary concept associated with the term "addiction" is wider than that proposed in AD. My aim, however, is not to capture our ordinary concept, but to refine it and make it useful for psychiatric and psychotherapeutic purposes. Refining the concept of ADDICTIVE DISORDER in the proposed way is fruitful because the presence or absence of tolerance and withdrawal makes a big difference for therapeutic purposes.

6.3.2 *Disorder versus Non-disorder*

AD clarifies what makes an addictive disorder specifically a *disorder*, and what makes it a *mental* disorder. In light of AD, the general picture is this: having a mental disorder (related to actions) is primarily a matter of conditions (i), (iii), and (iv) being met—an individual having the desire to φ, lacking the ability to omit φ-ing in view of their mental constitution and their life circumstances, and being harmed as a result of their φ-ing or their desire to φ. The fact that the ability is lacked in view of one's *mental* constitution (that is, one's relatively stable attitudes sensitive to reasons) is what makes it a specifically *mental* disorder.

6.4 A Competing View

Sinnott-Armstrong and Pickard (2013, 862) define "addictive disorder" as follows:

ASAP   S has an addictive disorder if and only if

  i   S has a strong and habitual desire to φ;
  ii   S's desire to φ significantly reduces their ability to control φ-ing; and
  iii S's desire to φ leads to significant harm.

According to Sinnott-Armstrong and Pickard, the degrees of control and harm counting as "significant" are determined by "what is at stake in making a judgment about addiction" (2013, 860) in a certain context. In the following, I focus on their view of control.

  Sinnott-Armstrong and Pickard (2013, 856) focus on the ability to control φ-ing in terms of two conditionals:

CONT   S has the ability to control φ-ing (where φ is an action) if and only if it is true that,

  i   if S wanted overall to φ, then usually S would φ and
  ii   if S wanted overall not to φ, then usually S would not φ.[13]

On this view, S has the ability to control playing golf if and only if S usually plays golf in situations in which they want to play golf and usually does not play golf in situations in which they do not want to play golf. The relevant ability here is the ability to control *whether or not* to play golf. The definition states "usually" because "occasional lapses do not prove lack of control" (Sinnott-Armstrong and Pickard 2013, 857). Sinnott-Armstrong and Pickard's example is that one might fail to play golf when one overall wants to "because the only golf course is closed or their car breaks down or they miss their starting time" (2013, 857). The definition states "overall" because desires can conflict with one another, and there may be a stronger desire to do something else. In such cases, not playing golf does not indicate a lack of control.

In the following, I will argue that CONT and ASAP are problematic:

1 *Flawed View of Abilities*: CONT rests on a flawed view of what it means to have an ability (to control whether) to φ in the first place.
2 *Insufficient View of Addictive Disorder*: ASAP is insufficient as an explication of what it is to have an addictive disorder.

Let me elaborate on each of these problems in turn.

1 *Flawed View of Abilities*
Conditional analyses of abilities, of which CONT is a version, have been widely criticized.[14] I point to one problem of CONT that is particularly relevant in the field of addictive disorder, namely impeded intentions.

A common objection against views like CONT is that they fail to account for individuals who lack the ability to form the overall desire to φ to begin with (see Lehrer 1968). Recall Betty, the golfer in a coma. There is a good sense in which Betty "cannot" control whether to play golf, because she cannot form the overall desire to play golf to begin with. The conditional analysis cannot capture these inabilities because it is true that *if* she wanted overall to play golf, she usually would play golf, and *if* she wanted overall not to play golf, she usually would not play golf (but then she wouldn't be in a coma). The conditional analysis cannot capture certain cases of inability; cases in which the individual lacks the ability to form the overall desire to φ to begin with.

In the context of addictive disorder, there is a related problem. Imagine an individual with an addictive disorder whose problem can be traced to an inability to form the overall desire not to φ to begin with. It might still be true to say that, (1) *if* they overall wanted to φ, they would usually φ, and (2) *if* they overall wanted *not* to φ, they would usually *not* φ. In these cases, CONT yields incorrectly that the individual has the ability to control whether to φ and hence that they do not have an addictive disorder. But because the individual lacks the ability to form the overall desire not to φ to begin with, clearly there is a sense in which they do not have the ability to control whether to φ, a sense that remains uncaptured by CONT.

2   *Insufficient View of Addictive Disorder*
ASAP proves insufficient for defining "addictive disorder" because (a) it cannot demarcate addictive disorder from other similar types of mental disorders such as OCD, and (b) it cannot differentiate disorder from non-disorder.

a   *Demarcation from Other Similar Types of Mental Disorder*
Consider an individual with an OCD related to handwashing. They have a strong and habitual desire to wash their hands (in response to particular internal stimuli such as obsessive thoughts), reduced control over this action, and suffer from their condition. Because they meet all conditions of ASAP, the analysis yields that they have an addictive disorder. However, both the *DSM-5* (APA 2013, 235) and the *ICD-11* (WHO 2019, F42) do not consider OCD to be a subtype of addictive disorder but rather a different type of mental disorder. Hence, ASAP is too broad to capture the actual use of "addictive disorder" as it pertains to the psychiatric and psychotherapeutic context.

Sinnott-Armstrong and Pickard might reply that their definition is revisionary. They state that the aim is to offer a theoretical definition, which does not require capturing the whole range of actual uses of a term. However, this conflicts with one of their other aims, which is to offer a definition that helps establish prognosis and indicate a treatment (see Sinnott-Armstrong and Pickard 2013, 853). Sinnott-Armstrong and Pickard (2013, 854) criticize that the *DSM* conditions for addictive disorder are too broad. But the *DSM* conditions are more specific than their own definition and presumably a broader definition will be even less useful by their own standards.

b   *Demarcation from Non-disorder*
Consider a typical case of lovesickness. Sina and Tony have been in a long-term relationship, but then Sina falls in love with someone else and breaks up with Tony. Tony is devastated. Everything reminds him of Sina, and he cannot but contact her, either because he misses her, he is angry at her, or he is trying to "win her back." Tony meets all conditions of ASAP. He has a strong and habitual desire to contact Sina and reduced control over his action to contact Sina. He is suffering. Hence, ASAP yields that Tony has an addictive disorder. In addition, it seems safe to say that breakups of long-term relationships typically cause suffering and reduced control of one's behavior. So, ASAP yields that typical cases of lovesickness are cases of addictive disorder. However, typical lovesickness is not considered pathological.[15] Hence, ASAP appears to be too broad to capture the distinction between disorder and non-disorder.

Is AD better equipped to distinguish between pathological and non-pathological lovesickness? At first sight, it is not, because one could argue that a lovesick individual lacks the ability to omit contacting their former partner in view of their mental constitution. However, what ultimately matters in AD is an individual's ability to respond adequately to their available (apparent) reasons. And in the case of typical lovesickness, the individual's mental constitution is such that they can easily regain the ability to control their behavior after some period of time.

Why should we believe this? In cases of typical lovesickness, the individual has a normative reason to grieve. In the aforementioned example, Tony has suffered a significant loss. Furthermore, Tony has a reason to hold on to the relationship with Sina because it is valuable to him. But Tony also has a reason to let Sina go: she does not want to be with him anymore. The typical process of grief—which involves "pangs of grief" and other emotions—is responsive to these mixed reasons (see Section 5.1.5). In general, individuals experiencing the typical process of grief come to terms with their loss. Thus, the mere fact that an individual experiences the typical oscillating process of grief indicates that they can easily regain the ability to control their behavior after some period of time.

Ultimately, AD allows for a differentiated view. Depending on how narrow or wide one understands "mental constitution" to be, the lovesick will have (or lack) the ability to omit φ-ing. If we focus on the specific mental states that make up lovesickness, then it turns out that the lovesick typically cannot omit φ-ing. But, if we look at their mental constitution more broadly, then the lovesick, typically, can omit φ-ing. So, if "mental constitution" is understood very narrowly, typical lovesickness turns out to be a disorder. However, we should not understand "mental constitution" in such a narrow sense because lovesickness is a condition for which individuals typically have adequate coping mechanisms. If we understand it in a broader way, then AD yields correctly that lovesickness is not an addictive disorder.

6.5 Conclusion

In this chapter, I have proposed the following explication of ADDICTIVE DISORDER: an individual has an addictive disorder if and only if they lack the ability to omit φ-ing—where φ-ing is characterized by the potential to cause tolerance or withdrawal—in view of their mental constitution and their life circumstances, and they are harmed by their φ-ing or their desire to φ. In turn, the ability condition should be spelled out in terms of the Success View. This view allows us to capture the idea that individuals with an addictive disorder may have problems on different levels: (1) they may lack the ability to follow through with their intention to omit φ-ing, or (2) they may lack the ability to form the rational intention to omit φ-ing, or (3) they may lack the ability to judge that they have a decisive reason to omit φ-ing.

How we conceive of abilities is highly significant. The conditional analysis of abilities suggests the following: to have the ability to φ is one thing, but to be properly motivated to φ is something else. If one φs—once one is properly motivated to φ—one has the ability to φ. If one does not φ, even if it is true that one would φ if properly motivated, then this is not a problem of ability but "just" one of motivation. What this view overlooks—but the Success View does not—is that motivation itself is an ability. Of course, sometimes one has the ability to φ but just doesn't want to φ, but it is possible that one lacks the ability to φ precisely because one lacks the ability to motivate oneself to φ.

AD offers a differentiated, more nuanced perspective on the compulsion versus choice debate. It suggests that there isn't only one sense in which an individual "can" or "cannot" omit φ-ing but that there are multiple, diverse senses. According to this view, individuals with an addictive disorder truly "can" omit φ-ing in one sense (holding their mental constitution and the presence of certain incentives fixed), but in another sense, they truly "cannot" omit φ-ing (holding their mental constitution and their life circumstances in which the incentives are not always present fixed). This suggests that just because an individual can do something under specific circumstances, we cannot infer that they can also do it under other, very different circumstances. Rather than searching for an absolute answer to whether individuals with an addictive disorder can or cannot omit φ-ing, we should ask a different question: under what circumstances can the individual with an addictive disorder do what they cannot do right now given the way their life is going?

Finally, let me point out another interesting consequence of AD. According to AD, individuals with an addictive disorder lack a certain ability to omit φ-ing, an ability that individuals without an addictive disorder possess. However, AD does not imply that individuals without an addictive disorder have greater *control* over (or are better at resisting) their desires than individuals with an addictive disorder. This is because it is possible for an individual to have the ability to omit φ-ing in view of their mental constitution (such that they do not have an addictive disorder) simply because they do not have the desire to φ to begin with. In this case, the ability to resist one's desire to φ is not exercised. For instance, if I do not have the desire to smoke today, it will be easy for me to follow through with my intention not to smoke today; there is simply nothing for me to resist. Contrast this with a scenario in which I do have the desire to smoke but successfully resist that temptation.

In light of AD, it is possible that there are individuals without an addictive disorder where the only thing that distinguishes them from individuals with an addictive disorder is that they do not have the desire to φ to begin with. We could say that these individuals, however, have a disposition to incur an addictive disorder in the following sense: they would not have the ability to omit φ-ing if they were to have the desire to φ. In sum, according to AD, individuals with an addictive disorder are bad at resisting temptation, but AD does not imply that individuals without an addictive disorder are any better at it. Perhaps, an addict lies dormant in us all.

Notes

1 Parts of this chapter draw on Dembić (2021).

2 For clarification, AD does not require that the individual experiences *actual* tolerance or withdrawal, but only that the φ-ing has the *potential* to cause them.

3 For a definition of ADDICTIVE DISORDER as a "strong appetite," see Foddy and Savulescu (2010). For critique of this view, see Sinnott-Armstrong and Pickard (2013). For influential theories of the causes and sustaining factors of addictive motivation, see Ainslie (2000) and Orford (2001).

4 Understanding "desire" in this wider sense ensures that at least some non-human animals qualify as proper subjects of addictive disorder. For creatures that do not possess desires, condition (1) would have to be adapted minimally: S engages in φ-ing recurrently and sufficiently frequently.

5 For a nuanced view on the value substance use has for an addict, see Pickard (2020).

6 See also Robinson and Berridge (1993), as well as Verheul, van den Brink, and Geerlings (1999).

7 Even in the ordinary sense of "being addicted to" this does not seem to be quite correct because "being addicted to breathing" sounds awkward, whereas "being dependent on breathing" does not.

8 On a phenomenological level, OCD and addictive disorder differ (see APA 2013, 235 and 481). This suggests distinct underlying structures (see Berger 2015, 251 and 484), although this is currently only a hypothesis. If it turned out that OCD and addictive disorders have more in common than initially assumed, the classification may change.

9 See Alegría, Bernardi, and Blanco (2010) and el-Guebaly et al. (2012), who compare gambling to paradigm cases of addictive disorder and OCD. Because this is an empirical condition, there is a caveat: depending on future empirical insights, condition (2) will have to be adapted accordingly.

10 See World Health Organization, "Withdrawal state" in: https://www.who.int/substance_abuse/terminology/withdrawal/en/ (accessed February 28, 2019).

11 Recall that the RHA is an explication of the concept of MENTAL DISORDER for scientific *and* normative purposes (see Section 1.2). The explication of ADDICTIVE DISORDER presented in this chapter is also one that aims to serve both types of purpose. This explains the necessity of harm (see Section 5.5).

12 This draws on Wallace's (1999) idea that addicts have an impaired ability to act in accordance with their own deliberative conclusion.

13 I reformulate Sinnott-Armstrong and Pickard's (2013, 856) view by using subjunctive rather than indicative conditionals to prevent misinterpreting them as material conditionals.

14   Some of the major problems include the following:

1   The truth of the conditional is not sufficient for having an ability (see Moore 1912; Chisholm 1966, 1976; Lehrer 1968; van Inwagen 1983; Wolf 1990; Whittle 2010; and Jaster 2020).

2   The truth of the conditional is not necessary for having an ability (see Johnston 1992, Fara 2005, and Jaster 2020).

3   The conditional analysis fails to elucidate the distinction between general and specific abilities (see Jaster 2020, 52 ff.)

4   The conditional analysis fails to account for degrees of abilities (see Jaster 2020, 55 ff.).

15   The claim is not that lovesickness or grief are never pathological. Although grief can certainly become a disorder (see APA 2013, 790), the claim is that in the *typical* case, lovesickness and grief are not pathological.

References

Ainslie, George. 2000. "A Research-Based Theory of Addictive Motivation." *Law and Philosophy* 19 (1): 77–115.

Alegría, Analucía, Silvia Bernardi, and Carlos Blanco. 2010. "Pathological Gambling: Obsessive-Compulsive Disorder or Behavioral Addiction?" *Revista Colombiana de Psiquiatría* 39: 133–142.

American Psychiatric Association (APA). 2013. *Diagnostic and Statistical Manual of Mental Disorders: DSM-5.* Arlington: American Psychiatric Association.

Berger, Mathias, ed. 2015. *Psychische Erkrankungen. Klinik und Therapie* (5th edn). Munich: Elsevier.

Chisholm, Roderick M. 1966. "Freedom and Action." In *Freedom and Determinism*, edited by Keith Lehrer, 11–44. New York: Random House.

———. 1976. *Person and Object: A Metaphysical Study.* La Salle: Open Court.

Dembić, Sanja. 2021. "Defining Addictive Disorder – Abilities Reconsidered." *Philosophers' Imprint* 21 (24): 1–23.

El-Guebaly, Nady, Tanya Mudry, Joseph Zohar, Hermano Tavares, and Marc N. Potenza. 2012. "Compulsive Features in Behavioural Addictions: The Case of Pathological Gambling." *Addiction* 107 (10): 1726–1734.

Fara, Michael. 2005. "Dispositions and Habituals." *Noûs* 39, no. 1: 43–82.

Foddy, Bennett, and Julian Savulescu. 2010. "A Liberal Account of Addiction." *Philosophy, Psychiatry, and Psychology* 17 (1): 1–2.

Heinz, Andreas. 2014. *Der Begriff der psychischen Krankheit.* Berlin: Suhrkamp.

———. 2017. "Der sich und Andere versuchende Mensch (Abhängigkeit)." In *Irren ist menschlich. Lehrbuch der Psychiatrie und Psychotherapie*, edited by Klaus Dörner, Ursula Plog, Thomas Bock, Peter Brieger, Andreas Heinz, and Frank Wendt, 361–423. Cologne: Psychiatrie Verlag.

Heinz, Andreas, and Anil Batra. 2003. *Neurobiologie der Alkohol- und Nikotinabhängigkeit.* Stuttgart: Kohlhammer.

Heinz, Andreas, Anil Batra, Norbert Scherbaum, and Euphrosyne Gouzoulis-Mayfrank. 2012. *Neurobiologie der Abhängigkeit.* Stuttgart: Kohlhammer.

Heyman, Gene M. 2009. *Addiction: A Disorder of Choice.* Cambridge, MA: Harvard University Press.

Hübl, Philipp. 2010. *Action and Consciousness.* Humboldt Universität zu Berlin.

Jaster, Romy. 2020. *Agents' Abilities.* Berlin: De Gruyter.

Johnston, Mark. 1992. "How to Speak of the Colors." *Philosophical Studies* 68 (3): 221–263.

Lehrer, Keith. 1968. "Cans without Ifs." *Analysis* 29 (1): 29–32.

Moore, George E. 1912. *Ethics.* Oxford: Oxford University Press.

Orford, Jim. 2001. "Addiction as Excessive Appetite." *Addiction* 96 (1): 15–31.

Pickard, Hanna. 2020. "Addiction and the Self." *Noûs* 55 (4): 1–20.

Robinson, Terry E., and Kent C. Berridge. 1993. "The Neural Basis of Drug Craving: An Incentive-Sensitization Theory of Addiction." *Brain Research Reviews* 18 (3): 247–291.

Sinnott-Armstrong, Walter, and Hanna Pickard. 2013. "What Is Addiction?" In *The Oxford Handbook of Philosophy of Psychiatry*, edited by William, K. M. Fulford, Martin Davies, Richard Gipps, George Graham, John Sadler, Giovanni Stanghellini, and Tim Thornton, 851–865. Oxford: Oxford University Press.

van Inwagen, Peter. 1983. *An Essay on Free Will.* Oxford: Oxford University Press.

Verheul, Roel, Wim van den Brink, and Peter Geerlings. 1999. "A Three-Pathway Psychobiological Model of Craving for Alcohol." *Alcohol and Alcoholism* 34 (2): 197–222.

Wallace, R. Jay. 1999. "Addiction as Defect of the Will: Some Philosophical Reflections." *Law and Philosophy* 18 (6): 621–654.

Whittle, Anne. 2010. "Dispositional Abilities." *Philosophers' Imprint* 10 (12): 1–23.

Wolf, Susan. 1990. *Freedom within Reason.* New York: Oxford University Press.

World Health Organization (WHO). 2019. *International Classification of Diseases 11th Edition* (ICD-11). Geneva: World Health Organization.

Conclusion

In the Introduction, I stated that Nives did not merely have serious "problems in living" (Szasz 1960). Rather, she was "not OK" in a mental health-related sense. My aim in this book has been to spell out this sense in more detail. More specifically, my aim was to provide an explication of the technical concept associated with the term "mental disorder" for both theoretical and practical purposes.

I proposed the following explication of MENTAL DISORDER (for the clearest cases that should fall under that concept):

RHA_{PSY} An individual S has a mental disorder if and only if

  i S does not have the ability to respond adequately to some of their available (apparent) reasons for (or against) some of their reason-sensitive attitudes or actions; *in view of* their mental constitution and their life circumstances (where the threshold of inability is determined by the degree at which individuals in the relevant comparison class are, on average, harmed by their condition C in some respect X), and

  ii S is harmed by their condition C in some respect X, *where X is some component of what makes S's life a non-instrumentally good one for S.*

In light of RHA_{PSY}, one could argue that Nives was "not OK" in the sense that (1) she was unable to cope with (some of) her "problems in living" in view of her mental constitution and her life circumstances and (2) she was harmed by the condition underlying or resulting from that inability in some relevant respects.

Before concluding, I wish to emphasize a few things that RHA_{PSY} does *not* imply.

First, RHA_{PSY} does not imply that the relevant ability is lacked completely. It is only diminished to a sufficient degree. Furthermore, it does not

DOI: 10.4324/9781003367840-8

imply that an individual with a mental disorder lacks all abilities to respond adequately to their available (apparent) reasons for (or against) their reason-sensitive attitudes or actions. It is only necessary that the affected individual has a "local" inability. However, the severity of the individual's mental disorder depends, among other things, on how "local" or "global" the relevant inabilities are.

Second, RHA_{PSY} does not imply that individuals with mental disorders have lives that are, all things considered, not "good enough." It implies only that the affected individual is harmed by their condition in some relevant respect X, where X is some component of what makes S's life a noninstrumentally good one for S.

Third, RHA_{PSY} implies neither that an individual with a mental disorder "cannot change" nor that they necessarily need help from others to change in a way to rid themselves of the mental disorder. Though an individual with a mental disorder lacks a mental disorder-relevant ability to φ in view of their mental constitution and their life circumstances, they may still have the ability to *learn* to φ in view of their mental constitution and their life circumstances and, thus, to change in a way to overcome their mental disorder (possibly even on their own).

Let me now draw two conclusions, a theoretical and a practical one.

First, RHA_{PSY} suggests that debates about whether those who have a mental disorder, "can" or "cannot" do otherwise are futile. There is simply no absolute answer here. RHA_{PSY} nonetheless suggests that there is, at least, one sense in which individuals with a mental disorder "cannot do otherwise." However, there might be many other senses in which they "can do otherwise." So, the more interesting questions to ask are "in which senses can they do otherwise?" and "in which senses can they not do otherwise?" Rather than focusing on a simple yes/no answer, we should identify the range of the abilities that individuals do and do not have when they have a mental disorder.

Second, RHA_{PSY} suggests that psychiatric treatment and psychotherapy could be about (1) *enabling* individuals with mental disorders to cope with their "problems in living" and/or (2) relieving the *harm* they are subjected to by their inability. Because the harm is tied to the inability, merely reducing harm without enabling the individual does not "cure" the mental disorder. Furthermore, sometimes, one can enable an individual (or the individual can enable themselves) by changing their external circumstances (for example, by removing social barriers or by ending a stressful relationship or job). This is not a new insight. RHA_{PSY} nonetheless provides a theoretical framework that renders intelligible why we can and should take such an approach to therapy.

Let me point out one important topic for further research. If we accept RHA_{PSY}, then assessing whether an individual has a mental disorder involves assessing whether they have a certain modal property—namely, an inability to φ. But, how do we know whether someone *lacks* the ability to φ in the relevant sense? Obviously, we cannot infer from the fact that they did not φ that they cannot φ. But what else could give us evidence for the lack of an ability? It seems that we need an epistemology of inabilities, an epistemology that can be utilized in the context of mental disorder.

Finally, I would like to emphasize that nothing in RHA$_{PSY}$ suggests that we should take what Peter Strawson (1962) would call a "managerial" view on individuals with a mental disorder. That is, we should not assume that we have to manage their lives for them because they cannot help themselves at all. It is only rarely the case that an individual with a mental disorder cannot cope with their problems *at all* (and some people even recover from their mental disorder on their own). Most often, enabling someone is about strengthening what is already there. It is about increasing their "degrees of freedom," as Wolfgang Blankenburg (1984) would say. It is likely that individuals do the best they can to cope with their problems. At least, I wish to believe that Nives did the best she could and that if she could have escaped her condition, then she would have chosen to do so.

References

Blankenburg, Wolfgang. 1984. "Prolegomena to a Psychopathology of Freedom." In *The Changing Reality of Modern Man*, edited by Dreyer Kruger, 174–190. Cape Town: Juta & Co. Ltd.

Strawson, Peter F. 1962. "Freedom and Resentment." *Proceedings of the British Academy*, 48, 187–211.

Szasz, Thomas S. 1960. "The Myth of Mental Illness." *American Psychologist* 15: 113–118.

Index

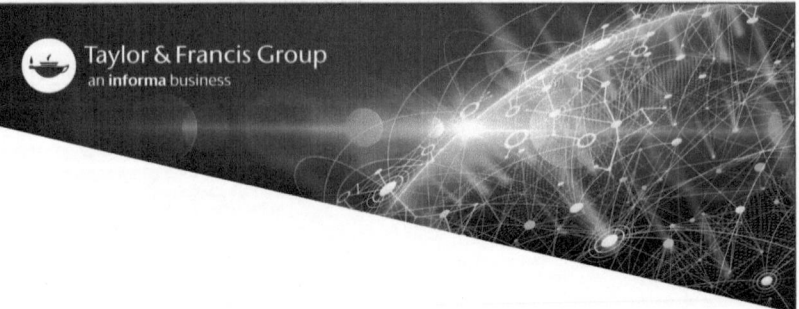
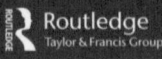
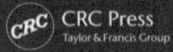